D1240424

FIRST AID

HOMOEOPATHY

in

ACCIDENTS and AILMENTS

by

D. M. GIBSON
M.B., B.S. (Lond.), F.R.C.S. (Edin.), F.F.Hom.

Sixteenth Edition 1993
ISBN No. 0-946717-10-9

Published by

The British Homoeopathic Association,
27A Devonshire Street, London, W1N 1RJ 071-935-2163

Table of Contents

First-Aid Treatment by Homœopathy

ACCIDENTS and AILMENTS

PROMPT homœopathic treatment in the earliest stages of illness and accidents will often avert prolonged suffering and serious disability. Effective treatment in established disease will speed up recovery and shorten convalescence. In both these respects homœopathy has proved of great value.

Apart from the obvious benefit to the patient, the burden is eased at home for the harassed mother, absence from class and games is lessened at school, and a great saving of man-hours is effected by diminished absenteeism through sickness.

The investigation and treatment of established disease should, of course, be in the hands of fully qualified physicians. But prompt aid is often called for in cases of illness or accident in home, school, office, factory and other spheres of activity, such as travel and sport.

Such aid can, as a rule, be most effectively supplied by homœopathy, and without the risks inseparable from the employment of many of the "popular" modern drugs, which carry risk of causing serious side-effects.

The mere fact that a drug is "the very latest" is no guarantee either of its efficiency or its safety. Nor is it reasonable to conclude that a remedy which was effective in former years should by the mere passage of time have become inert and useless.

That which is in accord with the laws of nature and assists life processes, be it food substance, air content or medicine, remains good for all time. It is for this very reason that homœopathy has withstood the test of time, and continues to prove a method of therapy valued greatly by physician and patient alike.

Accidents usually contain an element of surprise and take the victim unawares. These unfortunate events should not, however, catch us unprepared. Prompt action is usually called for and, if well-informed and wisely carried out, may make all the difference both at the time and also in relation to subsequent recovery.

It is essential to be well-informed as to the right and the best thing to do. Well-intentioned but misguided activities may do more harm than good, and it is in relation to this danger that there is undoubted aptness in the aphorism: "It is often better to do nothing than to do your best".

1

Wise instructions and due warnings may be found in many excellent books on "First-aid". It is not proposed to enter into what is more or less common knowledge, but to point out the very great contribution that homœopathy is able to make in the matter of recovery from accidents of various kinds.

Long experience has proved the value of certain remedies in relation to all manner of accidents for the purpose of countering shock, allaying pain, arresting bleeding, preventing infection and speeding convalescence.

The remedy of first importance in all types of injury is ARNICA, especially in the presence of shock caused either by the severity of the damage to tissues or by the emotional upset associated with the accident. One or two doses of ARNICA 200, spaced 15 minutes to half an hour apart, should always be given. Further measures are best considered in connection with the various types of accident which may occur.

EASY TO GIVE : RAPID EFFECT
Attention to Principles

Remedies used homœopathically are easy to administer and rapid in effect, but they must be used in accordance with the principles of the art and with due attention to right method of dosage. Harm can be done by the indiscriminate use of "homœopathic remedies", especially when the higher potencies are employed.

Only one remedy should be given at a time, and only a limited number of doses, enough to bring about relief. The doses also must be adequately spaced, the shortness of the interval between successive doses being in direct relation to the urgency of the situation.

For the sake of simplicity and to avoid confusion the potencies recommended are the 6c, 30c and 200c. A much wider range of potencies is available but the three selected cover the main indications in the circumstances under review. They are to be used only as directed.

Thus the 200c will be given as a single dose, or, perhaps, repeated once; the 30c will be limited to a few doses, about three to nine, spaced four to six hours apart in acute illness, or given twice or three times a day in less acute conditions; the 6c may on occasion be continued, twice or thrice daily, for a longer period.

Always the guiding rule is to stop the administration of the remedy when relief is obtained. The prolonged use of a remedy will defeat its own purpose by over-stimulation. Moreover, any drug administered for a prolonged period will be liable to induce a drug-disease with its own symptoms, causing in other words an "accidental proving". On occasion more harm can be done by over-medication and over-activity than by doing nothing at all.

The potencies suggested can be given in the form of medicated granules, pills or tablets. A few granules, or a pill or tablet, should be placed on or under the tongue and allowed to dissolve in the mouth. Tablets and pills, if hard, may need to be chewed. On occasion a good plan is to dissolve a few granules, say ten to twenty, or a tablet in half a tumbler of water and take a mouthful every half to one hour.

The emergencies and ailments dealt with are those in which prompt treatment can be given along homœopathic lines with good hope of benefit. Warning is also sounded as to what should not be attempted and against delay in seeking expert professional advice when this is called for. The manual is in no sense a medical treatise and matters of general medical interest, calling for expert attention and care, are not included.

A fuller explanation of the practice of this branch of medicine is given in a short textbook,"The Elements of Homœopathy," by Dr. D. M. Gibson. Published by the British Homœopathic Association.

Care Needed in Handling Homœopathic Remedies

HOMŒOPATHIC medicines require special handling and storage so that they may not lose their power and become inert as a result of contamination.

They should always be kept in the container in which they are supplied and never transferred to any other box, or bottle, etc. which has contained other substances.

They should be kept away from strong light, from great heat and especially from exposure to strong odours or perfumes, for example, camphor, menthol, moth balls, carbolic soap.

If stocks of remedies are kept in corked or screw top phials or bottles it is important never to uncork or uncover more than one remedy at a time. Neglect of this precaution would entail the risk of cross-potentisation and spoiling of the remedies.

Also the container should be uncorked or unstoppered for the minimum time required and care taken not to allow contamination of the cork or cap before replacement.

The medicines are usually supplied in the form of pills, tablets or powders. The dose should be tipped on to the clean palm and transferred to the mouth, or, if in powder form, be tipped direct on to the tongue. If more pills or tablets than the prescribed dose are shaken out of the bottle they must on no account be returned to the container, but should be thrown away. To put them back would risk contaminating the remainder.

No Need to "Wash it Down"

No water need be taken to "wash the medicine down". Absorption takes place from the mouth.

Sometimes the remedy is needed to be taken in water. The cup, glass, or spoon used should be "cleansed", before further use with another remedy. This is best accomplished by dry heat, the heat of an oven for, say, half an hour.

The dose should be put into a "clean mouth". It should not be taken until the mouth is free from the effects of food, drink, tobacco smoke, toothpaste, mouth washes and confectionery. An interval of half an hour should suffice.

While taking homœopathic remedies the use of all other crude medicines should be avoided, including laxatives, nasal drops and liniments. These may interfere with the action of the homœopathic remedy and destroy its effectiveness.

To ensure freedom from the risk of contamination at source the remedies should always be obtained from a reliable homœopathic chemist or from pharmacists who are prepared to take the precautions necessary to prevent the potencies from coming into contact with crude drugs.

———

Taken from "A Guide to Homœopathy", an introduction to this rational art of healing, published by the British Homœopathic Association,

Accidents

Contused Wounds

This type of injury is caused by the impact of or a knock against some hard blunt object with resulting damage to the soft tissues beneath the skin. In certain regions where the skin is close to bone, as in the head or over the shin bone, such a blow may split the skin causing a cut. But the main damage is to the tissues beneath the skin causing extravasation of blood and bruising. Pain, swelling and, later, many-hued discoloration result.

The possibility of serious damage to organs or of internal bleeding must be remembered, even though there is little sign of injury on the surface. This is especially so in connection with blows to the head, chest or abdomen. Increased pulse rate, pallor, distressed breathing, obvious deterioration in the general condition are danger signals which demand urgent skilled attention. Careful watch should always be kept for such signs when a severe blow has been sustained even though the immediate effects may seem to give no cause for alarm.

In this type of injury the immediate dose or doses of ARNICA 200 should be given, followed by ARNICA 30 three times or twice daily for a period, according to the severity of the damage. This will allay pain and promote the speedy absorption of the extravasated blood and greatly shorten the period of convalescence and disability.

If there seems to be delay in the disappearance of the bruise, and especially if the part remains cold and numb, it is a good plan to change to LEDUM 6 three times daily.

As always, when healing is well advanced, the medicine should be stopped.

A useful external application in contused wounds when the surface of the skin is unbroken is a compress moistened with ARNICA lotion (five drops of the mother tincture to the half pint of cold water). This must not be kept on too long as some skins are sensitive to ARNICA solutions, especially if applied too strong. It is the internal action of the remedy which is of greatest value.

Incised Wounds

The skin is cut by a sharp instrument which may have divided not only the skin but also the structures beneath the skin to a greater or lesser depth. A wound of this type will need careful surgical attention, especially if deep, or if gaping so that the edges cannot be drawn together without stitches. Even with a shallow wound in certain areas there may be divided tendons or nerves which have to be carefully identified and accurately sewn up. This is especially so in the fingers or at the wrist.

If the cut is superficial and no tendons are divided, as may be shown by the fact that all normal movements can be carried out, healing can be greatly facilitated by a HYPERICUM dressing. A little bleeding may be allowed, or even encouraged, to cleanse the wound from within outwards. A dressing of gauze or linen wrung out of CALENDULA or HYPERICUM lotion (ten drops of mother tincture to the half pint of water) should be placed over the cut and a bandage applied to help in stemming the bleeding and also in holding the edges of the wound together. If the wound is causing pain, a few doses of STAPHISAGRIA 30 can be given for relief.

Unless large blood vessels have been cut firm pressure will control bleeding, aided by elevation of the part if the wound is in a limb. A tourniquet is a most dangerous gadget and its unwise use has been responsible for innumerable disasters in the shape of gangrenous limbs, if not loss of life. Constriction must never be applied to a limb except in the case of uncontrollable spurting bleeding and then only as a temporary measure while expert assistance is being sought. If this is delayed the constriction must be released at half-hourly intervals and only reapplied if the bleeding recurs. A tourniquet must never be applied direct to the bare skin but over a pad of some soft substance (not too bulky). The same pressure that stops the bleeding will also interfere with the normal blood-supply to the limb and, if prolonged, gangrene (death of tissues) is only too likely to result.

In addition to the local dressing, CALENDULA 30 may be given internally twice daily to assist healing. The dressing must not be removed or interfered with but left in place till the wound has healed. It may well be kept moist the first day by dropping fresh lotion on the outside. This will aid in allowing serum to exude from the wound and not collect in a pool underneath it.

Dressings in General

It would be as well at this point to emphasise the all important fact that *dressings once applied to a wound should be left undisturbed for days*. At the outset the dressing can be freshly moistened from the outside with the lotion in use, but on no account should it be removed, or moved, even though it may be stained with discharge and become rather smelly.

It is realised now that the discharge of serum from a wound is part of nature's healing process and, moreover, that the freshly formed blood vessels and cells are extremely delicate and only too easily damaged by frequent changes of dressing accompanied by swabbings, irrigations and other forms of "messing about".

Not only do frequent dressings interfere with healing by causing damage to new blood vessels and growing cells but they involve pain and discomfort to the patient and, what is even more serious, the risk of fresh contamination of the wound by airborne germs in the dust of the room or ward.

Dressings should be left alone, firmly fixed with bandages to prevent movement and friction, until the wound is healed when they can be easily lifted away without causing bleeding or damage. Should there be evidence of local inflammation, in the shape of redness, heat, swelling and tenderness in the vicinity of the wound HEPAR SULPH. 6 should be given three times a day till these signs have subsided.

If there is a great deal of discharge the outer bandages and coverings can be changed and the skin around the wound cleansed with 75% alcohol, or with the lotion, taking care not to touch the edges or surface of the wound or interfere with the inner layer of dressings.

Lacerated Wounds

This type of wound is all too common in this modern world of speed and violence. Man's capacity for self-protection has lagged far behind his invention of potentially dangerous and destructive machines and gadgets of all kinds. As a result lacerated wounds are only too frequent.

In these wounds not only is the skin broken, but damage of greater or lesser severity is inflicted on muscles, nerves, blood vessels and other structures. The damaged tissues are often badly pulped and portions may be made non-viable and require surgical excision. Further, the wound is often contaminated by dirt or oil or clothing which has been driven into its depths.

Obviously such a wound requires skilled surgical attention with a minimum of delay, but as an immediate measure there will be no harm and every advantage in giving one or two doses of ARNICA 200 and in applying a first aid dressing moistened with HYPERICUM lotion (ten drops of mother tincture to the half pint of cold water) due attention being paid to control of bleeding as mentioned above.

In a wound of this type there is usually injury to nerves and HYPERICUM 6 should be given three times a day, especially if there are pains shooting centrally in the limb. If the pain is intense give HYPERICUM 30 every hour or so till relief is obtained. As a later follow up to speed healing, ARNICA 6 may be given twice daily for a shorter or longer period according to the extent of the damage.

Punctured Wounds

This type of wound is caused by a needle, nail, thorn, knife, splinter, or other sharp object. The wound in the skin may be insignificant, but deep structures may be injured with dire results or infection may be implanted deeply in the tissues, leading perhaps to the development of tetanus (lockjaw) if precautionary measures are not taken. Damage to important organs or large blood vessels is especially likely in punctured wounds of the chest or abdomen, and expert observation is called for in every case of a deeply penetrating wound even though the hole in the skin is quite small, and the wounded person inclined to make light of it.

The special homœopathic indication in wounds of this type is for LEDUM 30 internally, three times a day for two or three days. After this HYPERICUM 6 may be given, especially if the wound is painful or there are pains shooting up the limb.

On the other hand, should the part remain cold and numb or show sensitivity to touch, and relief be felt from exposure to cool air or from cold applications LEDUM should be continued in the 6 potency.

The danger of tetanus is especially present in punctured wounds owing to the fact that the tetanus bacillus is anœrobic, that is, can only multiply in the absence of oxygen. The risk of this serious complication is, of course, present also with other types of wound, and the prophylactic value of inoculation with tetanus toxoid is undoubted. In the event of injury a further dose of toxoid can be administered, obviating the need for anti-tetanus serum with its concomitant risk of serum reactions.

Scratches and Abrasions

These injuries are skin deep but in the case of an extensive abrasion a large area of skin may be denuded and possibly also ingrained with dirt or tar or other contaminant. Cleansing with cold water or CALENDULA lotion is called for and in some cases, especially if the face is involved, surgical attention under an anaesthetic may be needed to prevent subsequent disfigurement.

An endless procession of medicaments, highly vaunted antiseptics, brightly coloured dyes, liquid skin, tincture of iodine, ointments and salves have been employed at one time or another as first-aid dressings for this type of wound which, being superficial, is obviously extremely able to heal itself if given reasonable protection from interference and exposure to fresh contamination.

The ideal medicament for application to such a wound should be antiseptic, countering infection but not irritating the exposed raw surface; analgesic, allaying, not causing, pain and smarting; and above all non-toxic. CALENDULA and HYPERICUM in lotion or ointment form (ten drops of mother tincture to the half pint of water for the lotion) meet all these requirements ideally.

Many chemicals such as boric acid, carbolic acid, picric acid, if applied to an abrasion in liquid form carry a grave risk of causing poisoning as the result of absorption from the raw surface. They should never be used for this purpose.

Others, such as tincture of iodine or liquid skin applied to a raw surface cause most unpleasant smarting, and the former may be very irritating to iodine-sensitives.

CALENDULA and HYPERICUM have none of these disadvantages and should by no means be discarded in favour of one or other new-fangled "antiseptic" however loudly lauded and widely advertised by its manufacturers.

OTHER SPECIAL INJURIES

Bites and Stings

This type of injury presents an almost infinite variety, especially if overseas and tropical possibilities are included. In addition to the punctured wound inflicted, though sometimes, as in the case of a horse or human bite, the wound may be of the lacerated type, there is also an element of poisoning superadded. This may endanger life, as in the case of snake venoms, certain spider venoms, and so on. Even a bee sting may endanger life in a sensitive subject.

Apart from more serious effects the local irritation around a sting or bite may be most distressing and may lead to ulceration, especially if scratched.

Fortunately the remedy LEDUM is of very wide use in this connection. If the reaction is at all severe it would be wise to give one or two doses of LEDUM 200. In less severe reactions LEDUM 30 for a few doses, or 6 for more prolonged use, should suffice to reduce swelling, alleviate pain and counter the effects of the poison.

For a severe allergic reaction to bee stings CARBOLICUM ACIDUM 30 is advised, repeated every half to one hour or so at the outset if the symptoms are very urgent.

If there is much burning and stinging with rapid swelling of the part give APIS 30: if the part is very red, angry-looking, and burning give CANTHARIS 30: if the part affected is burning and blue in colour TARANTULA CUBENSIS 30 should give relief.

Coldness of the part with numbness or great sensitivity to touch and relief from cold applications, points clearly to LEDUM. If there are pains shooting up the limb HYPERICUM 30 or 6 would be the choice.

As an immediate external application to the bite or sting puncture a drop or two of the mother tincture can be dabbed on, thus:

for bee sting—LEDUM or URTICA URENS
for wasp sting—ARNICA or LEDUM
for gnat bite, etc.—CALENDULA or HYPERICUM
for snake bite—HYPERICUM

if the swelling persists the same remedies could be applied in lotion form as a compress.

In the event of a bite by a mad dog BELLADONNA 30, a dose every day for a week and then a weekly dose for the next six weeks, or LYSSIN 30, hydrophobia nosode, in similar dosage, should be of preventive value. However, in view of the fact that this appalling malady is fatal once it has developed, no delay should be lost in starting a course of Pasteur inoculations. While not neglecting this precaution of proven value, if available, it would certainly be wise to give also the recommended homœopathic remedy.

Certain other remedies are recommended in the event of the more venomous type of insect bite or of bites by snakes. Thus:

CARBOLICUM ACIDUM 30 patient appears comatose, with dusky face and pallor around the mouth:

CROTALUS HORRIDUS 6 rapid grave development of toxic symptoms, much local swelling with many-hued discoloration of the skin and effusion of dark blood from various sites:

ECHINACEA 6 parts septic or gangrenous, with foul-smelling discharge:

LACHESIS 30 much blueness of part and effusion of dark fluid blood:

OXALICUM ACIDUM 30 the colour is livid, parts cold and numb, with violent pains and tremors.

Needless to say the specially prepared antidotes related to the snakes found in any particular region should be used if available. The puncture wound should be sucked vigorously, and the venom spat out. This is a safe procedure provided that there is no crack or abrasion in lips or mouth. A ligature applied above the bite should not be so tight as to abolish the pulse below it. Both the limb and the patient should be kept at rest, and cool. First-aid measures to be of use must be applied without a moment's delay. Venom is very rapidly absorbed and efforts to prevent absorption are probably of little avail after about 10 minutes.

The ligature or tourniquet must of course not be left on too long, must not be applied over the bare skin, and must be released at half hourly intervals for a few seconds if a lengthy application is called for. In addition to these measures the internal administration of the appropriate homœopathic remedy should not be neglected. The more serious the condition of the patient the more frequently the dose should be repeated until there is improvement, when the interval between doses can be lengthened.

Fish stings inject a poison which is readily destroyed by potassium permanganate, a saturated solution of which should be injected into the wound or crystals rubbed in after incising the wound. Homœopathic remedies can be given as for snake bite.

Jelly fish stings should yield to APIS 30 or MEDUSA 30.

Burns and Scalds

Broadly speaking there are only two kinds of burns or scalds, namely slight and severe. All but the smallest burns must be regarded as serious and demanding skilled attention under strict aseptic surgical conditions. In fact a burn of extensive degree presents a most complex medico-surgical problem that can best be handled by a trained burn team in a modern hospital with up-to-date laboratory and other facilities.

There are three great dangers in burns or scalds. The first is **shock,** which is often grave because the psychological trauma of the experience is added to the actual physical injury. The second is **serum loss,** enormous quantities of fluid being poured out from the burned surface, thus depleting the body of vital proteins, salts and water. This results in interference with normal functions and increases shock. The third danger is that of **sepsis,** which is a later hazard and has caused many fatalities after apparent initial recovery.

Shock is inseparable from this type of injury. It is of vital importance in the first place not to increase shock by unwise activities and, in the second place, to counteract shock by relieving pain and preventing chilling. A dose of ARNICA 200 should be given at once, or of ACONITUM 200 if the patient is suffering from fright. This should be followed in a few minutes by CANTHARIS 30 to allay pain, a dose every 10 minutes or so till relief is obtained.

No burned clothing should be disturbed, but a dressing should be applied to cover any exposed burned area. Pieces of clean linen should be used for this purpose, either dry or wrung almost dry out of HYPERICUM lotion (ten drops of mother tincture to the half pint of water). The patient should be kept warmly covered in a well ventilated room. Overheating must be avoided as this would cause sweating and increase the danger of fluid loss.

IMPORTANT NOTE:—In the event of scalding with boiling liquid the saturated clothes must be removed as rapidly as possible and as gently as possible. The longer they are allowed to remain in contact with the skin the more serious the injury.

An immediate measure before the application of a protective dressing in the case of a scorch or a scald is to place the affected area of skin under the cold tap or in cold water. This helps to allay pain and also to diminish swelling.

An alternative to HYPERICUM is URTICA URENS, the remedy prepared from the small stinging nettle. The lotion (ten drops of mother tincture to the half pint of water) is an excellent dressing for small burns or scalds, or the ointment may be used. URTICA URENS 30 may be taken internally as an alternative to CANTHARIS for relief of pain. The dressing, of course, should not be disturbed once it has been applied, as explained above.

Numberless external medicaments have been recommended in the past for burns, including cod liver oil, tannic acid, various dyes, plain sterile gauze moistened with saline. A modern method of treating burns in hospital is to leave the cleansed burn area exposed to the air at a temperature of 65 to 70 deg. F. in order to encourage the formation by natural processes of a protective crust.

Picric acid was popular at one period but was found to carry the risk of toxic absorption with resulting damage to the kidneys. One useful emergency measure is to apply white of egg to the burned area. This is cooling and, if sufficient is applied, forms quite a good protective covering. But HYPERICUM or URTICA URENS have proved their worth and can be used with confidence.

Electric burns call for the same treatment as outlined above. Anti-shock measures are specially important.

Burns by chemicals present a special problem. The immediate need is to thoroughly sluice the contaminated skin with water.

Ear Injuries

Ears must be treated with great respect. It is most dangerous to poke into the ear with a match-stick, hairpin, or other object, on any pretext whatsoever. Not only may the lining of the canal be damaged but injury may be caused to the ear-drum with the consequent double danger of deafness and infection of the middle ear.

Nor is it advisable to put drops into the ear except under medical direction. Should the drum be perforated, instilling drops or syringing the ear would be likely to result in contamination of the middle ear with possible mastoid trouble as the outcome.

For the softening of wax in the ear a little warm oil can be run in on two or three consecutive days. The oil must, of course, never be heated over a flame, but poured into a spoon which has been warmed by placing it in hot water.

A foreign body may get into the ear canal by accident or be pushed in mischievously. This may be an insect, or a plug of wool, or some small object such as a bead or a pea. An attempt may be made at immediate removal by syringing with warm water (to which a few drops of CALENDULA or HYPERICUM tincture might well be added). A toy water pistol has on occasion proved useful for this purpose.

It is extremely important in syringing an ear not to use undue force and also to aim the stream upwards to impinge on the roof of the canal and not inwards towards the drum. If syringing, persisted in for some minutes, is not successful in dislodging the foreign body and washing it to the surface expert aid must be sought at once. Syringing should not be attempted if the drum is known to be perforated as may be the case if there is a history of ear trouble with discharge.

Should the patient be in great distress and panicky, as may well be the case with a child or nervous adult, ACONITUM 200 should be given, or a dose or two of IGNATIA 200 to allay anxiety. Should pain persist HYPERICUM 30 could be given, a few doses. If operative removal of the foreign body is called for ARNICA 30 may be given twice a day for a few days to ease the path of recovery.

Eye Injuries

Eyes must be treated with even more respect than ears. The most expert and skilled attention is called for in almost any type of eye injury. As a temporary measure a moist pad of HYPERICUM lotion (ten drops of mother tincture to the half pint of cold water) may be placed over the eye and ARNICA 200 administered. If there is much pain this can be followed by HYPERICUM 6 in hourly doses till relief is obtained. An alternative remedy is ACONITUM, which has been called the Arnica of the eye; give a few doses in 30 potency.

If pain is felt in the eyeball SYMPHYTUM 6, PHYTOLACCA 6, or COLOCYNTHIS 6 may be given. Pain persisting for a long time after the injury may yield to ARNICA 30, twice daily for a few days.

If there is a speck of dust or other foreign body in the eye it should be bathed in HYPERICUM lotion (two drops to the eyebath of warm water). If after this the object is still felt to be present the lid may be everted and if the speck is visible an attempt should be made to wipe it off with a wisp of soft handkerchief dipped in the HYPERICUM lotion. If the object is firmly embedded and cannot be easily wiped off, expert aid must be sought without delay. For persisting pain or discomfort after removal of the object, the eye should be bathed with EUPHRASIA lotion (two drops of mother tincture to the eyebath) and EUPHRASIA 6 given internally. A very useful fluid for use as an eye-wash is an infusion of tea leaves, warm or cold as preferred.

In "black eye" the damage is mostly around the orbit and the pain and discoloration and swelling cause both distress and disfigurement. ARNICA 30 should be given hourly up to five or six doses, or, if relief is obtained by cool applications, LEDUM 30. Further treatment may be with ARNICA 6 or, if the eye is painful, with HYPERICUM 6.

A "pair of lovely black eyes", unless separately administered, may indicate a fracture of the base of the skull and immediate steps must be taken to obtain expert advice. ARNICA should of course be given, a dose or two of 200; and 30 or 6 to follow.

For quick control of bleeding in a "cut eye" apply firm pressure with a pad soaked in equal parts of CALENDULA tincture and cold water.

Fractures

When a bone is broken there will usually be obvious deformity, with shortening and angulation of the limb. Sometimes this is not seen, as when only one of two parallel bones is broken in the fore-arm or the leg, or in rib fractures. Sometimes the broken fragments are impacted into each other and this may obscure the nature of the injury as deformity will not be easily detected and the use of the limb may still be present. However in almost every case of fracture there will be pain, swelling, tenderness over the broken bone and some disability.

The utmost care and gentleness must be exercised in handling a broken limb or spine. It is imperative to avoid any movement of the broken fragments, or any forward bending of the spine, lest further damage accrue to muscles, nerves, blood vessels, or the spinal cord. It is far better to do nothing until expert help arrives than to do the wrong thing. First aid implies firm gentle traction and some form of support that will prevent any movement of the jagged ends of the fragments during transport to hospital.

In any case of this type of injury ARNICA 200 one or two doses should be given, followed by ARNICA 30 or LEDUM 30 two or three times a day for a few days to help in absorption of extravasated blood and reduction of swelling. As a further aid to firm union between the fragments SYMPHYTUM 6 should be given once a day for a week or two. This remedy has also proved of great value in cases of persistent non-union of a fracture with accompanying disability.

Frostbite

It is important to realise that this condition can occur at temperatures above freezing point when chilling is combined with wetting. Under these circumstances it is usually known as trench foot or immersion foot, but the underlying pathology is the same.

The cause of frostbite is undue chilling by severe degrees of cold, or lesser degrees of cold abetted by damp, wind, circulatory stagnation, deficient nutrition or oxygen lack. This latter is specially likely at high altitudes when climbing or flying.

The most important factor in prevention is proper clothing. Several layers are warmer than one thick one, because warmth lies chiefly in the air between the layers. Every effort should be made to keep clothes dry. Clothes and boots wet with sweat or otherwise must be dried at every opportunity. Movement is important to keep the blood circulating.

If feet or hands, nose or ears, become numb no time must be lost. The part must be gently warmed by placing it inside a companion's clothing near the skin. Any rubbing of the affected part is useless and dangerous. Above all excessive warmth must be avoided as it can only do harm by increasing the swelling. The part must be kept at rest, arm in a sling and no walking if the feet are affected.

The affected part should be wrapped in a sterile dressing. This could be wrung out of HYPERICUM lotion (ten drops of mother tincture to the half pint of boiled water) or HYPERICUM oil used, if available. The dressing should not be disturbed. Internally give LACHESIS 30 twice daily for a few days or, if swelling is marked with burning and stinging, give APIS 30 in the same way. The chief needs are for gentle warmth, avoidance of rubbing and movement, and prevention of sepsis. Skilled surgical attention must be sought at the earliest opportunity.

Head Injuries

Injuries to the head are unfortunately increasingly common in this motorised age. One danger not sufficiently emphasised in many manuals on first aid is that of death from the inhalation of vomit or blood. The victim of a head injury is often unconscious and head injuries are frequently followed by vomiting. There may also be bleeding inside the mouth or throat. It is of the utmost importance to prevent the accidental inhalation of either blood or vomited matter into the windpipe and lungs as this may have the direst consequences.

This is liable to happen if the injured person is allowed to lie on his back. No time, therefore, should be lost in gently turning the casualty on one side with the head down and the jaws propped open to ensure a clear airway and allow blood or vomit to run out of the mouth. This position must be maintained until the patient is safely passed over to expert surgical care.

Any injury to the head must be taken seriously, even if after such injury the patient is able to walk and makes no very great complaint. A period of quiet, preferably lying down, and of constant observation is called for, a watch being kept for alteration in pulse rate or in

16

respiration, inequality of pupils, onset of headache, episodes of vomiting, twitchings of muscles or dulling of consciousness. Expert opinion is essential for proper assessment of the patient's condition. Damage to the brain or blood vessels in the skull may necessitate urgent surgical intervention.

Immediately following the injury, whether loss of consciousness has occurred or not, give ARNICA 30 half-hourly for five or six doses. When the patient has regained consciousness other remedies may be needed. If there are signs of irritation within the skull, stiffness of neck muscles, dilated pupils, spasms or twitchings of muscles, mental confusion, give CICUTA 30 three times or twice a day till relief is obtained. If there is pain at the back of the head with great heaviness of the eyelids and tremulousness of limbs, give GELSEMIUM 30.

Should headache or other symptoms persist NATRUM SULPHURICUM 30 should be given. This remedy is also of proven value when there is a story of a head injury with concussion in the past, even the remote past, whether the present symptoms appear to have any connection with the traumatic episode or not. A few doses of the remedy may clear up the symptoms and restore health in a surprising way.

Spinal Injuries

The spine may be jarred or jolted by a fall and this may sometimes lead to rather persistent symptoms. To prevent such a result ARNICA 200 one or two doses should be given at the time of the accident; followed by HYPERICUM 30 two or three times daily for a few days.

Serious injury to the spine always demands examination by X-rays and skilled surgical care.

Sprains

Sudden twists and turns may wrench, disrupt, or damage ligaments or "pull" a muscle. This type of injury is quickly followed by local effusion of fluid, pain and disability. A word of caution here. Such an injury especially if the result of a fall and in the neighbourhood of a joint such as the wrist or ankle, may not be only a matter of damage to soft structures but involve also damage to bone. The temptation to pass it up as "only a sprain" must not be yielded to, but careful X-ray examination carried out to check the possible presence of a fracture.

As soon as possible after the accident ARNICA 30 should be given every hour for five or six doses. This should be followed by RHUS TOX. 6 two or three times a day till better.

If the injury is close to bone and the bone covering (periosteum) is damaged RUTA 6 is to be preferred. Should the joint in the neighbourhood of the injury become swollen and distended with fluid, and painful on least movement BRYONIA 30 should be given three times a day till the swelling has receded, after which RHUS TOX. 6 can be used to continue the treatment.

Should the affected part be cold and numb but feel better with cold applications and be worse for heat LEDUM 6 is the remedy. If the damage is purely in a muscle, there is bound to be internal bruising and ARNICA 6 would be the best remedy.

For local treatment, ARNICA lotion (five drops of the mother tincture to the half pint of cold water) should be applied as a moist compress and a firm bandage put on for support. The limb should also be elevated, but this is not to say that movement should be neglected. In fact in this type of injury, and in the absence of any fracture, early movement, especially of the neighbouring joint, is of the utmost importance to prevent stiffness and subsequent disability. Physiotherapy is also most helpful, if available and skilfully employed.

A chronic sprain with local tenderness over a muscle attachment and pain on certain movements may result from repeated slight strain, often occupational in origin and not noticed at the time as harmful. Some stressful movement is made so frequently that in the end local irritation and pain develop at the insertion of the muscle involved. RHUS TOX. 6 or RUTA 6 will help to put such an injury right but it is also necessary to identify the cause and to correct it by avoidance of the harmful movement.

Surgical and Dental Operations

These events hardly come under the category of accidents but they inevitably involve injury to the tissues and loss of blood. ARNICA 30 should always be given if possible both before and after the event. ACONITUM 30 may well be given to allay fear and apprehension before this type of ordeal, especially in the case of children or nervous adults. It is also of use afterwards if there is much restlessness and tendency to toss about.

CALENDULA lotion (ten drops of mother tincture to the half pint of water) should be used as a mouthwash after tooth extractions and HYPERICUM 30 given internally if there is much pain, instead of ARNICA.

OTHER EMERGENCIES

Asphyxia

Although the literal meaning of this word is "pulselessness" it has come to mean in common parlance a condition of oxygen lack due to interference with respiration. It is evidenced by irregular breathing and a slaty blue or purplish appearance of the skin due to the lack of oxygen in the blood.

The most usual cause of this condition is a mechanical obstruction to the passage of air through the windpipe, but it may be due to depression of the respiratory centre in the nervous system by toxins or drugs, or to chemical changes in the blood as in poisoning by gas or exhaust fumes.

Obviously in the case of mechanical obstruction any measures that can be taken to clear the air-way should be carried out without delay, the jaws should be propped open with a cork or other available prop, the head placed on one side to prevent the tongue sagging back, and artificial respiration carried out. This is especially urgent if breathing has actually ceased as, for instance, in asphyxia from drowning. If mouth to mouth respiration is the method adopted, the head should be bent well back to open the air-way. The procedure of artificial respiration however correctly and energetically carried out is useless unless the air-way is clear.

Homœopathic remedies may be of service in some of these cases in addition to the relevant mechanical aids:—

ANTIMONIUM TARTARICUM 30 every ten to fifteen minutes till improvement is apparent, especially when the patient is full of sticky phlegm which won't come up—is "drowning in his own secretions"; face blue, cold and covered with clammy sweat; constant quivering of chin and lower jaw; rattling respirations.

CARBO VEGETABILIS 200 for a dose or two, 30 for further doses, when the face is puffy, pale, bluish or mottled, covered with cold sweat, and there is very obvious air hunger and collapse.

LAUROCERASUS 200 or 30 when the face is blue and cold as in the "blue asphyxia" of the newly born, and the patient is gasping for breath and clutching at the heart.

OPIUM 200 or 30 when the breathing is irregular, noisy, with long pauses, and cheeks are billowed out with every expiration: face red, bloated, suffused with blood, hot; pupils contracted; patient stuporous or in a coma.

Should breathing be obstructed by a sudden severe swelling of the tongue, or of the throat, then APIS 200 or 30 would be the remedy to use.

All such cases, of course, demand expert attention as soon as possible, but the use of one or other of these remedies without delay will prove of the utmost value and may assist in saving life.

Collapse and Shock

These are essentially the same condition. The term shock is used more in connection with accidents and operations, and collapse in relation to more "medical" cases.

The underlying disturbance is a failure on the part of the circulation to return sufficient blood to the heart; this failure may be due to various causes, severe poisoning, severe fright, severe injury and so on.

The symptoms and signs of the condition, which may be grave and endanger life, are due to the circulatory disturbance and the consequent lack of oxygen supply to the nervous system and other tissues. Prominent among these signs are an ashy grey pallor, a cold clammy skin, falling temperature with rising pulse (though sometimes the pulse rate may not be rapid at first), increasing difficulty in feeling the pulse, restlessness, shallow respiration, and a horrible feeling of impending disaster. The condition may be associated with hæmorrhage, either external or internal, but may be present without any actual bleeding. The tissues, however, are deprived of their normal supply of blood and oxygen by the circulatory failure, and this has a similar effect to actual hæmorrhage.

Certain immediate measures should be carried out in cases of shock. The patient should be reassured and fear allayed. The correct posture is lying flat in bed without any pillow and with the foot of the bed raised. This will assist in restoring adequate blood supply to the all important vital nerve centres in the brain. Warm coverings and hot drinks, such as hot sweetened tea, are needed as cold will increase the severity of the collapse. But over-heating must be carefully avoided as it would lead to further loss of fluid by sweating, and thus still further embarrass the circulation and the heart. Also the room temperature should not be too high or the air too stuffy as oxygen and fresh air are paramount needs.

CAUTION:—in case of injury or burns and the prospect of early hospital treatment under an anæsthetic *no fluids whatever should be given by mouth.*

Homœopathic remedies are of value and may be life-saving in this condition:—

ACONITUM if fear is very marked, 200 for one or two doses, or 30 every hour till better.

ARNICA 200 or 30 when there has been injury or bleeding.

CARBO VEGETABILIS 200 or 30 when there is great hunger for air, desire to be fanned, coldness, especially of the knees, cold breath, and mental torpor.

VERATRUM ALBUM 200 or 30 when the skin is marble-cold and there are beads of cold sweat on the forehead.

Convulsions

Convulsive fits are always alarming but are not always, in the case of infants or small children, cause for alarm. In the very young a convulsion is easily precipitated by such causes as fright, teething, fever, infections, rickets.

Severe or recurring fits call for expert diagnosis and attention. Immediate aid can be rendered by appropriate homœopathic remedies on the basis of guiding symptoms thus:—

ACONITUM 200 for a dose or two, or 30 for repeated doses up to five or six at short intervals, till relief is obtained, if the fit is very definitely the result of a fright.

AETHUSA 30 when the fit is associated with drowsiness after vomiting or after stool, or with cholera infantum: pupils large and fixed: thumbs clenched; teeth clenched.

APIS 200 or 30 when the fits are made worse by a hot bath or heat in any form, and associated with stiffness of neck muscles and a "meningitic cry".

BELLADONNA 200 or 30 sudden onset of fit, accompanied by blazing hot visage, burning skin, big staring pupils, violent movements, and aggravation by exposure to cold, to light, or by least jolt or jar.

CAUSTICUM 30 when fit is brought on by fear, by being chilled or occurs during the night with icy coldness of body; fit accompanied by screams, gnashing of teeth, violent jerking of limbs.

CHAMOMILLA 30 when fit is caused by anger or associated with teething and much peevishness; one cheek pale one burning red; hot sweat on face and head; thumbs clenched in palms.

CINA 30 when fit is brought on by any upset or by being punished, or in association with intestinal worms; grits teeth, clenches thumbs, exhibits chewing movements of jaws; turns on to belly.

CUPRUM METALLICUM 30 very violent convulsions; fingers flexed, thumbs clenched, jaws clenched, violent jerks and spasms; face and lips go blue; appearance of death after the fit; between fits is spiteful, violent, weepy.

GLONOINUM 30 especially when fit is brought on by exposure to the sun; head hot and congested; face dusky red; pupils small; fingers and toes not flexed but spread apart.

HYOSCYAMUS 200 or 30 when fit is caused by fright, or by worms, or comes on after eating; sudden irregular startings and twitchings; angular movements; frothing at mouth; wild look.

IGNATIA 200 or 30 especially after emotional upset as from being punished; fits may occur in sleep; face deathly pale; twitchings start in face, then goes stiff all over; body cold; fixed staring look.

OPIUM 200 or 30 violent spasms, may bend body backwards; cause may be fright; pupils very small; face dark red, mottled; child kicks off covers; worse hot room or hot bath.

STRAMONIUM 200 or 30 very violent spasms; one side convulsed, the other paralysed; head jerked from pillow; is afraid of dark but made worse by bright light or by touch of liquid on lips.

VERATRUM ALBUM 30 with fit face is blue, body is cold as marble, with beads of cold sweat on brow.

ZINCUM 200 or 30 especially if convulsions occur in association with infectious fevers, or suppressed eruptions; much rolling of head from side to side; ceaseless fidgety movements of feet and legs; much jerking in sleep; child is very cross before the attack.

In the main, of course, any kind of fit or convulsion is not a problem for home treatment, but on occasions the above remedies according to individual indications may prove of service for urgent and immediate use.

While on the subject of convulsions reference may be made to *epileptiform fits*. These may be due to old head injuries, or to other causes inside the skull, or to that little-understood and unpredictable disease epilepsy. All such cases must, of course, be under professional care; homœopathy in the hands of an experienced physician trained in this branch of medicine has often proved most helpful in relation to both the severer and the less severe types of the malady.

The epileptic fit is usually preceded by an aura, that is some disturbance of sensation or some peculiar feeling that gives warning of the approach of a fit. This is not always the case and fits may occur at night in sleep without any warning. At the time of the fit the tongue may be pushed out and then bitten by a spasm of the jaw muscles. It is well, therefore, to try and prevent this by placing a gag of some sort between the teeth for the protection of the tongue. Frequently also during the fit the urinary bladder will be emptied. Sometimes there is frothing at the mouth. The fall may be so sudden that injury may be sustained or a burn. After the fit the patient may pass into a deep sleep and awake later without having been conscious of having an attack.

Fainting

Feeling faint, or actually "blacking out", is the result of a temporary depletion of blood supply to the brain and consequent oxygen lack in the parts of the brain which control consciousness.

The circulatory system in some people is more labile, that is capable of sudden alterations, than in others. In such individuals an emotional shock, the sight of blood, the receipt of bad news, anger, fear, a stuffy atmosphere, or other apparently harmless cause, may bring on a fainting attack.

The body tends to correct the error in the distribution of the blood in a few minutes and energetic measures undertaken to "bring the patient round" are more likely to prolong the faint than to speed recovery.

If warned by a queer feeling and dimness of vision the best plan is to sit down and have someone press the head down between the knees. This will often restore the circulation in the brain and prevent the faint. If consciousness has already been lost nothing should be done except to keep the patient horizontal, loosen the clothing, especially about the neck and provide as much fresh air as possible. For the latter purpose it is obviously important to prevent curious or well-wishing onlookers from crowding around the patient.

If fainting is accompanied by pallor, air-hunger and sudden weakness internal bleeding should be suspected and expert aid sought without delay. Frequent fainting also demands careful professional investigation as this may be due to a variety of causes; many of these will respond to skilled homœopathic treatment.

The following remedies can be used when there is some obvious cause for the fainting attack, and are best given in the 30c potency:—

From anger	VERATRUM ALBUM
From emotional upset	IGNATIA
From excitement	COFFEA IGNATIA PHOSPHORUS
From exertion	NUX MOSCHATA
From fright	ACONITUM GELSEMIUM OPIUM
From hot stuffy atmosphere	LACHESIS PULSATILLA SEPIA
From kneeling	SEPIA
From loss of blood	CHINA
From loss of sleep	COCCULUS
From sight of blood	NUX VOMICA
From sight of needles, etc.	SILICEA SPIGELIA
From severe pain	ACONITUM CHAMOMILLA VERATRUM ALBUM
From slight pain	HEPAR SULPHURIS
From strong odours	NUX VOMICA PHOSPHORUS
In morning or after a meal	NUX VOMICA PHOSPHORICUM ACIDUM

An isolated episode of fainting, therefore, calls for a minimum of interference at the time. Repeated attacks demand expert investigation and care.

Hæmorrhage

Sudden severe bleeding is always alarming. Moreover it calls for expert investigation as to the source and cause, and observation under adequate conditions in case blood transfusion or surgical intervention is necessary.

To allay fear and anxiety ACONITUM 200 or 30 should be given, one or two doses. Absolute rest must be insisted on: if transport is called for this should be by stretcher or by ambulance.

Certain remedies have been found to be effective in bleeding of various kinds and occasion may arise when they can be used with advantage :—

ACONITUM 30 with blood of cherry red colour, and accompanying panic, anguished restlessness and thirst for cold or iced water.

ARNICA 30 when there is bleeding from mucous membranes or spontaneous bruising—purpura; and after injury.

ARSENICUM ALBUM 30 if there is great restlessness, anxiety and marked exhaustion.

BELLADONNA 30 when blood is bright red and hot, and clots readily; head hot and face red; pulse full and bounding.

BRYONIA 30 when blood is dark and fluid; there is nausea and faintness, made worse by attempting to sit up, and headache WORSE least movement.

CARBO VEGETABILIS 30 when the bleeding is associated with symptoms of collapse, coldness of face, breath, tongue, legs and feet, clammy sweat and great desire for air. There is a steady seepage of dark blood.

CHINA 30 when the hæmorrhage is associated with faintness, dimness of vision, ringing in ears and great weakness. There is a steady flow of darkish, almost brown, blood. Indicated in post-partum hæmorrhage.

CROTALUS HORRIDUS 30 when the blood is very dark, almost black, and remains fluid.

FERRUM PHOSPHORICUM 30 when the blood is bright red, clots readily, and flow is profuse.

HAMAMELIS 30 when there is a slow steady flow or persistent oozing of dark blood; exhaustion but no alarm or anxiety; bursting headache WORSE on stooping.

IPECACUANHA 30 when there is bleeding in gushes, bright red blood, associated severe nausea and dark bluish crescents below the eyes, gasping respiration, cold sweats on covered parts and weak pulse. Special indications are nose-bleed and hæmorrhage from uterus.

LACHESIS 30 when the blood remains fluid with flakes like little bits of charred straw; patient is WORSE from heat and averse from anything tight round waist or neck.

PHOSPHORUS 30 when the bleeding is bright red, in fits and starts, and persistent; feeling of emptiness and coldness in belly; thirst for cold drinks, or craving for ice or ice-cream. Often of value in bleeding from polyps, or from fibroid tumours of uterus, also when there is a tendency to spontaneous bruising.

SABINA 30 brisk flow of blood with dark clots, associated with pain extending from the pubic region backwards. Indicated in abortion.

SECALE CORNUTUM 30 with passive flow of dark offensive blood; patient is chilly but desires to be uncovered.

VERATRUM ALBUM 30 indicated in intestinal hæmorrhage accompanied by collapse, cold sweat on brow and air hunger.

A dose of the selected remedy should be given every ten minutes or so till the bleeding is controlled. *Brandy or other stimulants must on no account be given as the effect on the circulation would cause fresh or increased bleeding.*

Heatstroke

This is a serious condition brought on by exposure to high temperatures. High humidity of the atmosphere may be a contributory cause. There is profound failure of the heat regulating function, and progressive rise of temperature to a dangerously high level results. Other symptoms are circulatory collapse, cramps or convulsions, and coma. Warning symptoms are lassitude, headache, giddiness, nausea and diminution of sweating.

The attack may start with vomiting, muscular twitchings and convulsions. The skin is hot and dry, and both temperature and pulse rate are raised. There may be diarrhœa and scanty urine. Delirium, drowsiness or excitement give place to coma, and the issue may be fatal.

The most urgent need is to lower the very high temperature and this is best achieved by cold sponging and continuous fanning. If possible the patient should be in a cool room about 65 deg. F. and at a low humidity, or in a cool shady spot out of doors. The patient should not be left lying on the gound but placed on a table or a bed. The head should be kept high and constantly cooled. No time should be lost in thus reducing the temperature to a level of 101 deg. F.

Homœopathic remedies are of great value in this condition as accessory aids to recovery. Probably the most useful of these is GLONOINUM 6 or 30 a few doses at half hourly or hourly intervals till improvement is obvious. The indications for GLONOINUM are waves of terrible throbbing, bursting headache, hot flushed face, and sweaty skin. With dilated, fixed pupils, bounding pulse, burning hot dry skin, and delirium BELLADONNA would be the choice.

Severe cramps would call for CUPRUM METALLICUM. Splitting headache, WORSE least attempt to move, and nausea, WORSE trying to sit up, would suggest BRYONIA.

There is a tendency for the condition to relapse and it is advisable to keep the patient under supervision in cool surroundings for a few weeks after recovery. Poor ventilation, overcrowding, heavy clothing, debility, muscular fatigue, and alcohol are possible contributory factors, as is also an inability to perspire.

Nose Bleed

Spontaneous bleeding from the nose (*epistaxis*) is sometimes profuse and alarming. The bleeding is at times from small veins just inside the nostrils, and in this case firm pinching of the nose just behind the tip may help to stop the flow. It is, of course, useless to pinch the bony bridge further back.

Probably the best way to control the bleeding is to allow natural coagulation to take place and not allow this to be interfered with by swallowing movements which cause negative pressure and dislodge freshly formed clots. In order to achieve this end the patient should be propped up leaning forward or to one side and a large pad of cotton wool placed for the blood to trickle into from the nose. This will prevent backward flow into the throat with consequent swallowing. As a further measure a cork, or other prop, should be placed between the teeth and the patient instructed NOT to breathe through the nose and not to swallow. Blood from the nose or saliva from the mouth must be allowed to dribble on to the pad of wool. This procedure permits the clot in the nose at the bleeding point to become adherent and the bleeding will stop naturally. Should this method fail expert aid must be sought.

As adjuvants to natural control of the bleeding one or other homœopathic remedy should be given, q.v. section on hæmorrhage. Of special value in this connection is VIPERA 200 one or two doses. With profuse flow of bright red blood FERRUM PHOSPHORICUM 30 may be given for a few doses till bleeding has stopped.

Frequently recurring nose-bleeds will call for expert consultation as to the cause.

Panic and Fear

Fear is a symptom and a very unpleasant and distressing symptom at that. There may be an obvious cause for the feeling of fright, or terror, or panic, but quite often it seems to be quite irrational. None the less the fear itself is real enough at the time it is experienced.

Homœopathic remedies are of the greatest value in relation to this distressing, little understood, and not always sympathised-with symptom. The right remedy will allay the fear and replace it by calm, cheerfulness and confidence. One or two doses of the 200 potency or, perhaps, the 30 repeated for two or three doses, will usually suffice.

ACONITUM sudden fear or fright from definite cause, or "out of the blue"; desperate with fear; beside himself with fear; impatient, inappeasable, "something must be done, and quickly".

ARGENTUM NITRICUM fear and apprehension beforehand; stage-fright, exam funk; sudden panic in a crowd, in a closed space (tube train, lift, *et sic*), on a high place, or over water; dread of death.

ARSENICUM ALBUM sudden unaccountable fear, associated with unease and restlessness; intolerable anguish; sudden waves of fear when alone.

GELSEMIUM paralysed with fear; all of a dither; knees quiver; trembles all over; wants to be sat on or held firmly to control the shaking; especially before any ordeal.

OPIUM fear as the result of some shattering experience, and the fear persists.

STRAMONIUM fear in the dark or at sight of some glistening object.

Poisoning

Poisoning as an acute emergency may be suicidal, homicidal or accidental. Both suicidal and accidental poisonings are on the increase, the latter especially among children, who have too ready access to modern drugs of dangerous toxicity and prevalent use.

In acute poisoning prompt action is of vital importance. There is not a moment to lose. Time should not be lost from the immediate care of the patient by looking for clues or hunting up antidotes. The immediate need is for removal of the poison from the body or its neutralisation in the stomach.

The latter course must be pursued if the poison swallowed is corrosive, in which case there will be burns or stains on the lips and in the mouth and, possibly, confirmatory evidence in the shape of stains on the clothing or the floor, or the label on a bottle or other container beside the patient.

Corrosives are either strong acids, sulphuric, hydrochloric, nitric, or strong alkalis, caustic soda, caustic potash, ammonia. The neutralising agent must be given in sips, to prevent vomiting, and in large quantities to help dilute the poison. Up to a pint should be given for adults, less in the case of a child. Too much fluid must not be given for fear of distending and rupturing a stomach wall damaged by the corrosive substance ingested.

To neutralise the above acids use magnesia, four tablespoonfuls to the pint of water, or if this substance is not available one of the following may be used, chalk, whitening, washing soda, or soapsuds.

To neutralise alkalis give vinegar, six tablespoonfuls to the pint of water, or the juice of six lemons in the same quantity.

It should be noted that phenol (carbolic acid) and salts of lemon (oxalic acid) are mild corrosives and if one of these has been swallowed an emetic should be given and the stomach washed out.

Washing soda or bicarbonate of soda must not be used if oxalic acid or oxalates have been taken. Instead use magnesia, chalk, or rely on washing out the stomach.

In every case, except the swallowing of the above mentioned corrosives, the urgent need is to rid the body of the poison as quickly and as thoroughly as possible. The sooner gastric lavage can be carried out the better, and in summoning professional aid the probability of poisoning must be mentioned so that the apparatus for washing out the stomach will be brought and no time wasted.

The fact that the patient has already vomited, if this is the case, is no reason for delay in giving an emetic and, or, in washing out the stomach very thoroughly.

As emetic give warm salt and water, one tablespoonful of salt to half a tumbler of warm water. Force the patient to gulp this down quickly so as to encourage vomiting, and keep on till vomiting has occurred not once but many times.

Emetics cannot, of course, be given to an unconscious or comatose patient. In this case lavage must be carried out and in the prone, head-down, position to prevent backflow of fluid into the air passages and choking.

In cases of poisoning by mushrooms salt and water should not be given as this might lead to increased absorption. Mustard, one tablespoonful in half a tumbler of warm water, should be swallowed, and followed by copious draughts of warm water.

In this type of poisoning give AGARICUS 6 or 30 every 15 to 30 minutes till improvement is apparent.

Poisoning associated with severe vomiting and purging and extreme exhaustion with restlessness calls for ARSENICUM ALBUM in similar dosage. With similar symptoms but cold sweat on brow and collapse give VERATRUM ALBUM. In marked collapse with air hunger and desire to be fanned give CARBO VEGETABILIS. Should there be fiery burnings, burning pain on passing urine, and pallor of face CANTHARIS is indicated. With restless tossing and great fear a dose or two of ACONITUM would be called for.

Poisoning cases often manifest symptoms of shock and this should be dealt with as mentioned above in the section on collapse. Expert aid must always be sought in these cases. Also, when the immediate needs of the patient have been attended to, careful note should be taken of any evidence of the source of the poison (bottle, box of tablets, or other container), of any odour that has been obvious (in patient's breath or in the room), of any stains on clothing, bed-covers, etc., and any relevant details of the surroundings (bedside table, medicine cupboard, letter or note left by patient, and so on). Such details should not only be noted but written down at the time and given to the doctor to help in the diagnosis and subsequent handling of the case.

Stroke

This is the term usually employed in connection with what used to be called apoplexy. As the name implies there is frequently an element of suddenness about the event. A stroke is a vascular accident within the skull. One of two things may occur. Either the clotting of blood in a blood-vessel inside the skull causes throm-bosis and the sudden cutting off of the blood supply to a larger or smaller patch of brain, or a blood-vessel bursts and cerebral hæmorrhage causes damage to brain substance of a greater or lesser degree.

The immediate effect of such an accident may be slight or it may be catastrophic. In the case of lesser degree there will be a sudden attack of weakness in a limb, or in the muscles of speech, or a sudden numbness which persists, or sudden confusion of thought.

When such happenings as these occur, especially in an old person the main need is for complete rest in bed with reassurance. ACONITUM 30 should be given for a few doses to allay anxiety and engender calm, and then ARNICA 30 two or three times a day for a few days to encourage healing of the brain injury and absorption of extravasated blood. All such cases must, of course, be under expert medical care.

In the more severe case the patient may fall unconscious and in this case aid should be summoned at once. No attempt should be made to get the patient upstairs and into bed, but a mattress may be brought to the room and placed under the patient with due cover-ings to maintain warmth. A dose of ARNICA 200 may be slipped under the tongue and the head kept turned to one side to assist breathing and prevent saliva, or perhaps vomit, getting into the air passages. As such an accident is an alarming experience for those in attendance a dose or two of ACONITUM may be indicated for them. It will be a great help to the doctor when he comes to find every one calm and able to describe exactly what has happened.

In a comatose patient with dusky, flushed face, noisy breathing puffing the cheeks out at each expiration, OPIUM 30 is the remedy of choice.

29

Ailments

Abscess and Inflammation

An abscess is the result of successful action on the part of the defences of the body in dealing with an intruder. Infection occurs somewhere in the tissues, implanted by a contaminated weapon or other instrument, entering through a scratch or through damaged or unhealthy skin, or conveyed to the site involved by the blood or the lymph.

The presence of infection rouses the defences of the body to mobilise their resources and hurry them to the scene of action. Large numbers of white blood cells are called up and much serum is poured out at the infected spot. The main job of the white cells is to deal with germs, ingest them, digest them, and thus put them out of action. The serum not only dilutes the poisons present but also brings auxiliary aid in the shape of antitoxins and other defence factors.

This vital defence reaction is associated with and implemented by a greatly increased supply of blood to the part. This together with the outpouring of fluid into the tissues results in the well-known symptoms of inflammation, viz. heat, redness, swelling, pain and tenderness.

If the defence reaction is fully successful the invader may be scotched and repelled without further to do, but more often it is a question of containment and localisation with abscess formation. The content of the abscess is the pooled collection of serum with dead white cells, for many die in the process, and other debris of battle. This fluid is called pus; it is shut off from the surrounding tissues by a newly formed wall of fibrous tissue.

The treatment of an abscess is, of course, a matter calling for surgical experience and skill. What then has homœopathy to contribute in this connection? Certain remedies can be of very great value both in the early stage of inflammation, and also in the later stages of the episode, to speed up healing of the tissues and restore the status quo. Given early according to the symptoms the remedies may even prevent the formation of an abscess and bring about speedy resolution of the inflammatory process.

The following remedies may be indicated in inflammatory conditions (a few doses of 30 potency at 4 hourly intervals, or 6 potency three times daily till better):

APIS MELLIFICA shiny, swollen appearance ; pains which sting and burn; WORSE heat in any form; may jerk awake with pain at night; absence of thirst.

ARNICA deep inflammation with much soreness, blueness of part; aversion from being touched; bed feels hard.

30

ARSENICUM ALBUM burning and stabbing pains, relieved by heat; great restlessness of mind and body; thirsty for sips; WORSE soon after midnight.

BELLADONNA tense, bright red swelling; affected part burning hot and throbbing; parts very tender to touch; thirst for small amounts of cold water; feverish, with large pupils; WORSE exposure to cold air or least draught.

CROTALUS HORRIDUS grave illness accompanying septic infection; tendency to bleeding from mucous surfaces; skin cold, dry, mottled; "blood-poisoning".

FERRUM PHOSPHORICUM early inflammation, symptoms of mild degree.

GUNPOWDER which is a mixture of nitre with sulphur and charcoal, is a valuable remedy in septic conditions. It is usually prescribed in the 3x potency.

HEPAR SULPHURIS easy suppuration from least scratch; pains sharp and stabbing; parts excessively tender to touch; patient extremely sensitive to touch, pain, people, surroundings; irritable, cross, peevish; WORSE cold in any form; wants to be warmly wrapped.

LACHESIS parts look blue or purplish; aversion from least touch or constriction; is cold and clammy; WORSE from heat and after sleep; anxious, restless, suspicious, loquacious.

PYROGENIUM inflammation accompanied by violent chills; hot and cold; restless to an extreme degree; rapid pulse with low temperature; gravely ill.

SILICEA inflammation of rather slow development, often affecting deep tissues or lymph nodes; chronic septic conditions; helps in recovery after an abscess or other inflammatory episode.

Anæmia

There are several varieties of anæmia. It is essential for the diagnosis of anæmia that a proper examination of the blood be carried out. This diagnosis is often made on altogether insufficient evidence; and wholly unnecessary, even harmful, treatment may be given as the result. This is inexcusable.

Homœopathic remedies are indicated in certain forms of anæmia, but must be prescribed under the guidance of a homœopathic physician who has access to laboratory facilities to check progress.

Appendicitis

This condition is, of course, one for immediate reference to expert opinion. It should be pointed out, however, that every pain in the belly is not due to appendicitis, and also that inflammation of the appendix may occur without some of the usual common signs.

The best plan is to regard severe pain in the abdomen as always something to refer to the doctor, and *never on any account to be treated by the administration of castor oil, or any other purgative.*

Should the services of a doctor for any reason be unobtainable the patient should be put to bed, kept at rest, and nothing but sips of water given by the mouth.

The appendix is a small, short tube leading off from the caecum or first part of the large bowel. It may become inflamed in a catarrhal manner and in this case the inflammation will tend to resolve on rest and careful diet. But, on the other hand, the tube may become obstructed and shut off from the general bowel cavity. This is a very grave and very urgent complication and immediate surgical advice and intervention is imperative. The inflamed and obstructed organ will "blow up", perforate or become gangrenous, sometimes in a matter of hours.

In the event of professional aid being unobtainable the rest treatment may be supplemented by one of the remedies mentioned as being helpful in inflammatory conditions, q.v. Abscess. Among these LACHESIS has been found useful when pain is felt in the right, lower quadrant of the abdomen.

Asthma

This is a highly individual affliction. It is important, if at all possible, to be under the care of a homœopathic physician as the adequate treatment of the condition requires intimate knowledge of the homœopathic materia medica and also of the homœopathic art. Most so-called "cures" for asthma are no more than muscle relaxants and give temporary relief to the spasm of the bronchial tubes. Moreover the substances used in these sprays and tablets are often quite toxic or irritant in themselves. Homœopathy on the other hand is capable of providing not only temporary, but also lasting, relief to sufferers from this most distressing malady.

Bilious Attacks

There is much nausea, sensation of sickness, often accompanied by loathing for food, frequent vomiting of green or yellow bile-stained fluid, and much exhaustion, even to the point of prostration.

Rest in bed, warmth, and rest to the stomach are the main requirements. Probably nothing by mouth is best, but thirst may be relieved by sips of water, glucose or orange juice. Bovril or chicken broth may be acceptable later on.

Homœopathic remedies will help (a few doses of 30 or 6 till relief is obtained):

BRYONIA especially when there is accompanying headache, and when the least attempt to move or to sit up intensifies the symptoms; thirst for large quantities of fluid, not cold, at long intervals; dryness of mouth and lips.

COCCULUS attack brought on by anger, grief, chagrin; nausea intensified by thought, sight or smell of food; inclination to vomit accompanied by profuse salivation; better lying flat and keeping quiet.

IPECACUANHA nausea and vomiting, both severe and persistent; nausea not relieved by vomiting; abundant flow of watery saliva; attack may follow over-indulgence in rich food; tongue remains clean; shivery and shudders; but WORSE either extreme of temperature.

KALI BICHROMICUM nausea and vomiting in alcoholics; stomach upset by mildest food; symptoms accompanied by blinding headache; yellow vomit.

NUX VOMICA aftermath of over-indulgence; nausea and vomiting; much retching and gagging; tongue like leather; foul taste in mouth; queasy nausea in morning; unduly irritable.

A severe attack, or recurring attacks, must be referred to a physician for adequate investigation, assessment and treatment.

Bladder Trouble

Inflammation of the bladder will require medical investigation and care. In an emergency, when there is much frequency in passing water and burning pain and discomfort, a few doses of CANTHARIS 6 may give relief.

Blood Pressure

This term signifies a blood pressure that is above the usual level. Some people get on quite happily with a blood pressure that is "high" by accepted standards. Others in good health have a pressure that is "low" by comparison with the average level. In fact it is often a chance discovery that a blood pressure is "high" or "low", and in the absence of associated symptoms such a finding has probably not much significance and should not be allowed to cause alarm. It is most important that such anxiety be avoided, as worry and apprehension are in themselves factors which tend to raise the pressure.

If the blood pressure is unduly raised and other symptoms are present it goes without saying that physical and emotional strain and stress must be carefully guarded against. Worry must not be indulged in and weight must be kept down. Alcohol and tobacco should be avoided. Exercise out of doors within reasonable limit s is to be encouraged. With regard to drug treatment one fashionable depressor of blood pressure follows another, but most of these are drastic in action and not free from risk of unpleasant side-effects.

The health of the individual as a whole must be attended to and mere pre-occupation with the blood pressure alone is an ill-advised approach. The homœopathic method has, therefore, much to offer in this condition under the guidance of a doctor.

Boils

A boil results from septic infection of a hair follicle or one of the other numerous pits in the skin. The intense reaction in this limited space produces a conical swelling which at first itches and then becomes extremely painful owing to the great tension within the swelling. There is no greater mistake than to squeeze a boil. Such treatment is not only painful but tends to spread the infection to the surrounding tissues.

A boil must be covered, for protection, either by a plain clean dressing of lint or gauze or by a small compress wrung almost dry out of HYPERICUM lotion (ten drops of tincture to the half pint of water) and left alone.   Nature will deal with the situation and in due course produce a core of dead tissue in the centre of the boil with a little fluid pus.   This will come away in the dressing when the boil has softened.   At this stage a fresh dressing may be applied and the surrounding skin cleansed with HYPERICUM lotion or with surgical spirit.

Homœopathic remedies are of the greatest value in assisting the healing process.   The remedies referred to above under "Abscess" will apply in some cases, but two remedies are of special significance in relation to the treatment of boils.   With very acute inflammation, severe pain, burning, stinging and throbbing TARANTULA CUBENSIS (30 for a few doses, or 6 for a few days) is indicated.   Another remedy of great value in similar cases, especially if there is blueness or blistering and an exceedingly angry appearance of the inflamed area, with a black centre is ANTHRACINUM 30.

Chronic or frequently recurring boils will present a problem for the homœopathic physician to deal with.

Carbuncle

A carbuncle is an area of septic inflammation below the skin and in this way differs from a boil which is definitely in the skin.   This is more serious as the opportunity for the inflammatory process to spread in all directions is much greater and septic absorption is more likely to occur.   Thus a large area may be involved, with the production of a raised plateau-like swelling as distinct from the cone-shaped swelling of a boil.   Sooner or later the overlying skin will become inflamed too and break down in spots, which show up yellow in the purplish affected skin, and discharge pus.

A carbuncle is a more serious affair than a boil and expert medical care will be called for, not only in the matter of treatment, but also in the investigation of any general systemic disease that may be present, such as diabetes mellitus. Treatment formerly was in the main surgical, but more conservative methods are now employed. As in the case of boils the "similar remedy" will be effective, notably ANTHRACINUM, TARANTULA CUBENSIS, or LACHESIS.

Chicken-pox

Although this malady may present a very constant symptom picture, yet from the point of view of homœopathic treatment the constitutional or temperamental aspects of the case must also be taken into account. On occasion chicken-pox may be mistaken for small-pox, or vice versa. This might be disastrous and expert knowledge is required to avoid such an error of judgment.

An undoubted case of chicken-pox can be helped by such remedies as the following (a few doses of 30, or 6 for more prolonged administration, two or three times daily):

ANTIMONIUM CRUDUM child peevish, cries if looked at, touched or washed.

ANTIMONIUM TARTARICUM pustules are very large; child peevish and whining, wants company.

PULSATILLA child mild and tearful, and not thirsty.

RHUS TOXICODENDRON great restlessness of mind and body.

SULPHUR (two or three doses) hungry but eats little, extremely thirsty.

If desired, contacts may be given RHUS TOX. 30 three doses during a 24 hour period, by way of prevention.

Chilblains

A chilblain is a vascular accident. An originally rather sluggish circulation in an exposed part, at a distance from the central cardiac pump, is further slowed down and stagnated by cold. As a result the local blood-vessels become engorged, their walls damaged and distended, and leakage of serum occurs. This produces the well-known symptoms of local redness, swelling, itching or burning.

This condition once established tends to right itself as soon as the weather warms up, but exposure to radiant heat, proximity to the fire, can only increase the leakage of serum and make matters worse.

Prevention is of the greatest importance; protection from undue chilling is essential both indoors and out. One exposure to undue cold can do damage which will take weeks to put right. Warmth of hands and feet must not be sacrified on the altar of fashion in hosiery or footwear. Gloves should be loose-fitting and warm. Ears should be protected in very cold weather.

Homœopathic remedies will help recovery when chilblains have occurred. As treatment may have to be continued for a period the lower potencies, e.g. 6c, should be used:

AGARICUS much burning, itching, marked redness, WORSE when cold.

CALCAREA CARBONICA the feet especially are damp and cold; *RELIEF* from cold.

NUX VOMICA in thin, tense, irritable patient who hates wind.

PETROLEUM much burning and itching, with cracks, chaps and split finger tips.

PULSATILLA condition WORSE from heat and from letting limb hang down; patient craves air, may be tearful or irritable.

As external applications the mother tincture of TAMUS COMMUNIS or CALENDULA may be painted on, or either RUTA ointment or TAMUS ointment rubbed on.

Cholera

This dread disease may be mentioned in case prompt action should be called for overseas in an area where cholera is common and, possibly, efficient medical aid scarce.

An individual in apparent health is suddenly struck down and seized by the most violent symptoms of vomiting, diarrhœa and cramps. Rapid dehydration results and death may occur in a few hours.

Prevention is of the greatest moment. The chief essential is that everything eaten or drunk should be thoroughly cooked or boiled. Raw vegetables, salads, and fruit, melons included, must on no account be eaten. Scrupulous cleanliness must be insisted on, both in personal hygiene and in the kitchen.

Three remedies are especially to be thought of in this disease (one or two doses of 200, or 30 every quarter to half hour till improvement sets in):

CAMPHORA extreme degree of prostration, surface icy cold, complains of burning in abdomen, with desire to be uncovered.

CUPRUM METALLICUM cramps very marked, icy cold all over, wants to be covered, not sweating.

VERATRUM ALBUM drenching cold sweats, especially on brow, marble coldness of surface, violent diarrhœa and vomiting.

Colds

Much time, money and ingenuity have been expended in the search for the "cause" of "the common cold". At one period this was said to be a germ, Micrococcus Catarrhalis. At the present time the "causal factor" is one or more of several viruses. It is probably nearer the truth to say that the common cold is not a specific illness with a single cause, but a certain kind of response to a combination or variety of causes.

Faced with a certain set of circumstances one person will develop a cold. Another person faced with the same set of circumstances will not. This is because one of the most important factors in this adverse situation is the response of the individual. If an individual has good resistance, immunity, or whatever it is, his response to the circumstances that "give" someone else a cold will leave him un-scathed. It is, therefore, this internal protection, or susceptibility as the case may be, that will be the deciding factor in "catching a cold" or in not catching it, or being caught by it.

This is where homœopathy comes in most helpfully, because homœopathic treatment enhances resistance to infection and other hostile factors as well as assisting in the cure of established disease. A greatly diminished susceptibility to colds has often been recorded in the experience of those who are having, or have been having, homœopathic treatment for other reasons. Moreover, when a cold is contracted, homœopathic remedies carefully matched with the existing symptoms will often speed the cure and cut down the period of convalescence and disability.

A liability to constant colds calls for careful investigation by a homœopathic physician. A cold already "caught" will tend to be self-limiting; recovery will be speedier if it is possible to stay indoors, in bed if feverish, and keep warm and out of draughts. Many homœopathic remedies are of service in this connection, prescribed according to the principle of similars, a dose or two of 200, 30 repeated four-hourly for a day or two, or 6 three times a day, till relief is obtained. Sometimes in the course of clearing up a cold the symptoms may alter and a further remedy be called for on this account. Some of the possible remedies are mentioned below :

ACONITUM to be given at the first sneeze, or first shiver, especially after exposure to dry cold; frequent sneezing, with dropping of clear hot water from nostrils; fever, thirst, restless at night, buzzing in ears; WORSE in stuffy atmosphere.

ALLIUM CEPA paroxysms of sneezing, eyes and nose stream, nose and lip become sore and raw; hot, thirsty, headachy; WORSE in warm room, *BETTER* in fresh air; rawness may extend to throat and chest.

ARSENICUM ALBUM takes cold with every change of weather; sneezing frequent and painful, thin watery, burning discharge, which makes lip sore, or is stuffed up especially at night; an intense tickle inside the nose at one particular spot; tends to spread to chest; extremely chilly; sensation of "ice cold water or, maybe, boiling water, coursing through veins"; thirst for small amounts of water.

BELLADONNA very violent onset after exposure, especially of head, to chilling; not much discharge, nose swollen, sore, red, hot; throat raw, sore, hoarse; flushed, hot, with violent headache; very thirsty.

BRYONIA onset is delayed, and symptoms slow in developing; much sneezing, eyes red and water, nasal discharge is watery; lips and mouth are dry and there is great thirst for large quantities; tendency to spread to chest with painful cough, and severe headache; *BETTER* when lying down and keeping perfectly still.

DULCAMARA when cold follows exposure to cold wet weather, or becoming chilled when over-heated; sneezing is severe, WORSE in a cold room; wants nose kept warm; eyes are red and sore; eyes and nose both stream, especially indoors and in a warm room; neck stiff, throat sore, pains in back and limbs.

FERRUM PHOS. 30 is recommended for use in the early stage of a cold without very marked indications.

GELSEMIUM the influenza type of cold; from warm moist weather, or from change in weather; discharge makes nostrils sore; chills up and down spine; hot and cold by turns; headache with heavy feeling in lids and limbs; tearing tickling cough, which is *BETTER* near the fire.

HEPAR SULPHURIS follows exposure to cold, dry weather; affects nose, ears, throat, chest; much sneezing, especially in cold wind; discharge at first watery, then becomes thick, yellow and offensive; nose swollen and painful; WORSE from least draught, or even putting hands or feet out of bed; must be well wrapped up; peevish and hypersensitive.

KALI IODATUM colds from every exposure, especially to damp; violent sneezing; watery acrid discharge; eyes smart and water severely; nose red and swollen; frontal headache or pain at root of nose; face red; hot and cold by turns; violent thirst; WORSE from heat.

MERCURIUS sneezes violently; nose drips; fluent, corrosive, greenish-yellow, offensive discharge; nose red, swollen, shiny, sore; throat often sore and voice hoarse; dry, tickly cough WORSE both extremes of temperature; pale, flabby, indented tongue; foul taste in mouth; profuse sweats and feels no better after; starts with creeping chilliness.

NUX VOMICA from exposure to dry cold; much sneezing; nose alternately blocked or running, stuffed up at night, streams in warm room and daytime, rather *BETTER* out of doors; extremely chilly, can't get warm, shudders after drinking fluids or from least movement; cold and hot by turns; fits of sneezing after meals; mouth dry; excessively irritable.

38

PHOSPHORUS begins in chest or throat; sneezing which causes pain in throat or head; nose alternately blocked or running, or one nostril blocked and the other discharging; often streaks of blood on handkerchief; nose red, shiny, sore; throat sore and voice hoarse; tight feeling in chest; racking cough WORSE going from warm room into cold air or vice versa.

PULSATILLA when cold is persistent; stuffed up at night or in warm room; otherwise thick, yellow, bland discharge, especially profuse out of doors; pains in face and nose; chills up and down back; possibly blood on handkerchief; loss of appetite, taste and smell; chapped, peeling lips; cheeks hot; feels *BETTER* out of doors and WORSE coming into warm room.

These are some of the remedies covering the variable symptom pictures presented at one time or another by "a cold".

Nasal drops and inhalants should be avoided. Not only would they counter and annul the homœopathic remedy, but their constant use probably tends to prolong the unhealthy state of the membranes lining nose and throat. The frequent forceful shrinking of the mucus membranes by drug action is calculated to have an irritant effect. Moreover the cure of disease must be from within outwards and the internal remedy is the all-important factor in this. Forceful suppression of symptoms by drastic drug action may interfere with natural cure and do more harm than good.

As a cold preventive it has been found of value to take a dose of BACILLINUM 30 once a month during the winter. A popular method is to combine with this INFLUENZINUM 30, given in one dose. This, it is claimed, affords added protection.

Colic

This type of pain is caused by violent contractions of the muscular walls of tubular organs such as the intestines, the bile ducts, and the ureters. The pain "doubles one up" and comes in spasms. Such pain calls for medical investigation as to causation and treatment. The immediate spasm may be relieved by one of the following remedies, a few doses of 30 or 6, given every quarter to half hour till better :

BELLADONNA especially when relief is obtained by bending forward.

BRYONIA the pain is made WORSE by least movement, jar, touch or pressure; also WORSE from heat; patient lies motionless on back with knees drawn up.

CHAMOMILLA belly blown up and wind passed in small quantities without relief; *BETTER* by application of local heat; colic of teething infants.

COLOCYNTHIS writhes and twists in pain; can't keep still ; some relief from hard pressure, also from passage of wind; attack may be associated with or brought on by emotional upset, especially anger.

MAGNESIA PHOSPHORICA *BETTER* by heat, pressure and walking about; not relieved by belching; infants lie, crying, with lower limbs drawn up and are soothed by application of warm hand.

NUX VOMICA from over-eating; *BETTER* when sitting or lying down.

Constipation

In this connection it is most important to realise that to insist on a bowel movement every day without fail is contrary to nature. Food taken in at the mouth is subjected to a lengthy process of disintegration by mechanical movement, as well as by chemical and bacterial activities. The nutritive elements are in this way made available for absorption and the residue is passed on down. This residue or bulk is essential for normal rhythmic bowel movement, and is ideally provided by a diet based on whole meal bread and foodstuffs which have not been tampered with, adulterated, or devitalised.

The end portion of the bowel, the so-called rectum, is normally empty, and while this is so no amount of straining can produce a bowel movement. In the normal natural course of events at some time or other during the day the contents of the large bowel will be propelled on down into the rectum with a resulting urge to stool. When this occurs—it may be once a day, more than once a day, or only once in several days—that is the time for the bowel to be emptied.

The main causes of constipation are civilisation and purgatives, or laxatives. It matters not whether the latter be herbal or synthetic, drastic or mild, they are contrary to nature and upset the balance and rhythm so essential to normal bowel action; and they often cause much griping and disturbance of digestion in other ways. The use of aluminium cooking utensils, kettles, coffee-pots and so on is thought by many to be a frequent cause of constipation and there is a good deal of evidence in confirmation of this theory.

An established condition of constipation may present a difficult and tedious problem calling for expert medical advice and guidance. The following are some of the remedies that may be indicated in this condition, (a few doses of 30, or more prolonged use of 6, unless otherwise mentioned):

ALUMINA absence of urge to stool; sits and strains till cold and trembling, and then passes a soft stool, or perhaps a lot of little balls, or very narrow stools.

BRYONIA mouth, tongue, lips all very dry; stools are dry, hard, black as if burnt; much thirst for large quantities of cold water; may be given as 1x tincture, three to five drops in water each morning.

HYDRASTIS stools hard, knotty, the fragments united by shreds of mucus; may feel nauseated about 11 a.m. and complain of empty faintness in stomach region; aversion from bread and vegetables; sallow complexion; give three to five drops of 1x tincture in water each morning.

NUX VOMICA much ineffectual urging to stool; even after passage of stool rectum does not feel properly emptied; too many laxatives taken in the past; tendency to bloating sensation; very chilly and maybe irritable.

OPIUM complete absence of urge to stool, perhaps for days on end; stools are composed of little hard balls; poor appetite; drowsy in daytime, sleepless at night with over-acute awareness of noises.

SILICEA constant ineffectual urge to stool; stools hard and may slip back when partially expelled; anus seems closed by spasm of its muscles.

SULPHUR frequent urge but inadequate evacuation; stools hard, dry, black and only expelled by great effort with pain and burning; alternation of constipation and diarrhœa.

Corns

These thickenings of the skin, with a central and exquisitely painful core, are usually due to the pressure of ill-fitting footwear or to faulty posture. Expert advice should be sought in these matters. Corns once formed can be pared, down to and including the hard white central core, with due care not to cause bleeding or invite infection. ANTIMONIUM CRUDUM 6 can be given to encourage softening and allay pain. RUTA ointment can be rubbed in, or VERATRUM VIRIDE mother tincture painted on to reduce surrounding inflammation.

Cough

A cough is usually the result of some form of irritation affecting the air passages, such as occurs with a "cold" or derives from habitual smoking. However, various other disturbances within the chest, some of them serious, may give rise to a cough, which is not a symptom to be lightly regarded or merely palliated with lozenges, linctus, or proprietary medicines.

The cough that accompanies a cold tends to clear up when the cold gets better. As a means of prevention, any obvious source of irritation in connection with the air breathed day by day must be tracked down and avoided as far as possible. In foggy weather it is wise to cover the nose and mouth with a scarf and thus reduce the quantity of soot and sulphur fumes breathed in. Having the windows open at night is of no advantage at all when the air so admitted is cold, polluted, and harmful to throat and lungs. When there is decent fresh air available the habit of deep breathing is of great value in preventing colds and coughs.

Inasmuch as a severe or constant cough may be associated with serious disease it is most important that expert aid be sought to discover the reason for the cough and to advise in the matter of treatment. Self-dosing with cough mixtures and the like is most unwise and may be dangerous by delaying diagnosis and proper treatment. The taking of homœopathic remedies without adequate investigation as to the true nature of the underlying trouble is equally to be condemned.

A recent cough of the catarrhal type may yield to one or other of the following remedies, a few doses of 30, two or three times during the 24 hours, or 6 for a few days, till better.

ACONITUM constant short, dry, cough with feeling of suffocation; or dry, hard, ringing cough; after exposure to cold, dry wind.

ANTIMONIUM TARTARICUM persistent cough with rattling respiration, great accumulation of sticky phlegm, and great difficulty in getting it up; sudden sensation of suffocation and must sit up; sunken, sickly, pale or bluish countenance.

ARSENICUM ALBUM wheezing respiration, much frothy phlegm; cannot breathe freely or fully; WORSE from midnight to about 2 a.m.; very restless and anxious; weak and exhausted to a marked degree.

BELLADONNA dry tickling cough in violent paroxysms; great dryness in larynx; cough seems to burst open the head; fit of coughing ends in sneezing, or a whoop; child begins to cry just before fit of coughing comes on.

BRYONIA hard, dry, spasmodic cough, which shakes the whole body; associated with stitches and soreness in chest, and with bursting headache; WORSE from cold, dry weather, especially east winds, at night, and after eating and drinking; wants to sigh, but deep breath hurts; WORSE any movement; peevish, wants to be let alone, thirsty for large drinks of cold water at long intervals, but hot drinks tend to help the actual cough. The sufferer holds on to both chest and head when coughing.

CAUSTICUM hard cough, racks whole chest, which seems full of mucus; rawness in throat and hoarseness of voice; inability to expectorate; swallows phlegm; may get relief from a drink of cold water. There may be loss of urine when coughing.

DROSERA violent tickle in larynx brings on a fit of coughing, which seems deep down in chest, and is accompanied by retching

42

and gagging; cough causes pain below ribs and calls for support by the hands; WORSE at night. Of proven value in whooping-cough. The cough tends to be better in the open air.

HEPAR SULPHURIS suffocative coughing spells, croup; WORSE in cold, dry weather, and when breathing cold air; aggravated by uncovering any part of body, even putting a hand out of bed; *BETTER* in warm, moist weather. The patient is chilly and sweaty, and is thirsty for hot drinks.

IPECACUANHA spasmodic, suffocative cough with rattling respiration early in illness; wheezing, with sensation of weight in chest; child may become blue and go stiff; intense nausea with clean tongue; nausea not relieved by vomiting.

KALI BICHROMICUM persistent cough, with very tough mucus which is lumpy or stringy; constant hawking.

NUX VOMICA dry teasing or spasmodic cough, with gagging and retching; feverish, but cannot move or uncover without feeling desperately chilly; cough causes bursting headache; WORSE cold, dry windy weather; oversensitive to least stimulus.

PHOSPHORUS dry, hard, tickling cough which racks the body and is very exhausting; the tickle is in the larynx or lower down; cough causes bursting headache; must hold chest when coughing on account of pain; tightness in chest; sense of weight or oppression in chest; WORSE any change in temperature, warm to cold or the reverse, on lying down at night, laughing, talking, eating, lying on left side; thirst for cold drinks, or iced water, which tends to be vomited when warmed in stomach.

PULSATILLA dry, teasing, persistent cough, possibly with spells of gagging and choking; aggravated by taking a breath; WORSE in warm room, in evening, when lying down, and interferes with sleep; desire for air and open windows; tearful, intolerant of heat, neither hungry nor thirsty.

RHUS TOXICODENDRON dry, teasing cough with tickle deep down in air tubes; WORSE at night, uncovering, even a hand, cold wet weather; taste of blood in mouth though no blood seen; very restless, must keep moving.

RUMEX spasmodic cough, dry or with tough, tenacious, stringy phlegm; paroxysms preceded by violent tickle in throat pit; WORSE breathing cold air, and covers mouth; hoarseness with constant desire to hawk; WORSE soon after lying down at night and on waking in a.m.; sensitive to open air. A curious feature is that, on breathing in, the inspired air feels cold.

SPONGIA noisy, rasping cough without wheezing or rattling; wakes from sleep choking, in great alarm and with violent cough; WORSE talking, singing, swallowing, lying with head low; may be tough phlegm, difficult to cough up and usually swallowed. Hot drinks afford relief, also taking food.

Cramp

Cramp is due to a violent spasm in one or more muscles, often in the calf or the sole of the foot, which is brought on by interference with the normal circulation of the part. Cramp may result from exercise or, conversely, from slowing of the bloodstream when lying in bed. Another common cause is excessive sweating, as in the cramps of miners and stokers, or dehydration from some other cause as in cholera.

Where the cause is obvious, preventive or curative measures must be employed accordingly. Incidental cramp will usually pass off in a few minutes, with the aid perhaps of massage or by stretching the contracted muscle. Constantly recurring cramps call for medical consultation, preferably homœopathic. A remedy often found useful is CALCAREA CARBONICA 30, night and morning for a week. In more severe cases CUPRUM METALLICUM 30 can be given in a similar manner.

CUPRUM ARSENICOSUM in 3x potency is often effective. It is recommended to take two tablets in the late afternoon, two early in the evening and two more at bedtime for prevention of cramp during the night. This dosage should not be exceeded as the remedy is a poisonous substance and the potency is low. Also the tablets should not be left lying about and accessible to children.

Croup

This alarming suffocative attack occurs in young children of two to four years of age. It is rare under six months. It usually happens at night, the child waking into a paroxysm of breathlessness characterised by crowing inspiration, barking, metallic cough, husky voice, violent struggles for breath and clutching at throat. Both child and parents are usually terrified; this tends to aggravate the spasm. The attack lasts half to three hours and then suddenly eases and the child settles off to sleep. Attacks are apt to recur for two or three nights. The child is usually already suffering from a teasing cough before the onset of the attacks.

Three remedies have been found of special value in this condition: ACONITUM, HEPAR SULPHURIS, and SPONGIA (q.v. preceding section on Cough). The most applicable one should be given every 2 hours or so (30 or 6, till relief is obtained, or at longer intervals to prevent recurrence of the attack).

Suffocative breathing which does not quickly pass off with relaxation of spasm must be investigated without delay as the cause may be diphtheria, the presence of a foreign body in the air-passages, or other pathological condition resulting in pressure in or on the wind-pipe. Sometimes sudden œdematous swelling of the larynx may threaten to choke the patient, and urgent tracheotomy may be called for. In this condition there is also usually obvious and severe swelling of the epiglottis at the back of the tongue; the remedy to give with the least possible delay would be APIS (200 for one or two doses, or 30 for several doses, at half to one hour intervals) while summoning expert aid.

Small children sometimes are seized by a sudden spasm of the larynx with cessation of breathing, rigidity of body, blueness of surface, and the worst seems about to happen. However the seizure terminates with a long crowing inspiration and the attack is over for the occasion. To expedite matters it is advised to sit the child up, slap its back, tickle its nose with a feather, throw cold water on its face or place a hot sponge on the outside of the throat.

A prompt dose of ACONITUM would probably be equally, if not more, effective. The attack may follow an emotional upset and occur during the night. The condition may be associated with rickets, and in any case of repeated attacks adequate medical investigation is called for.

Diarrhœa

Normally by the time the contents of the digestive tract reach the terminal portion, or rectum, they are no longer in a fluid state. Should the rate of downward propulsion be speeded up, or should the absorptive capacity of the bowel be diminished by disease the contents of the bowel will still be in a liquid state when they reach the rectum. Loose stools (or diarrhœa) will be the result.

This state of affairs is produced in various ways. Fear or undue anxiety and nervousness may so interfere with normal bowel rhythm as to greatly accelerate the rate of propulsion, and acute diarrhœa is the result. But other causes have a similar effect, notably the presence in the stomach or intestines of irritant matter, swallowed in food, manufactured in the bowel in disease or deliberately taken in the shape of laxatives. Most of these are herbal in origin and all of them provide an unnatural stimulus to bowel movement, the normal and healthy stimulus being that provided by a varied diet with plenty of bulk in the shape of roughage.

Interference with normal digestive processes by one cause or another, or actual disease of the bowel itself, may also result in abnormally fluid rectal contents; chronic diarrhœa will be the result. Such a condition must be adequately investigated and dealt with; it is not a problem for home medicine.

For simple, temporary or incidental attacks of diarrhœa several remedies are available (as usual a few doses of 30, or of 6, should suffice):

ACONITUM diarrhœa brought on by exposure to cold, dry wind or result of fright.

ALOE diarrhœa accompanied by colicky pains both before and at the time of stool; urgent call to stool soon after taking food or drink; sense of insecurity at anus. There is a constant urge to stool but only flatus may be passed, and perhaps urine at the same time. After passage of stool prostration is marked and accompanied by sweating from weakness.

ARNICA diarrhœa complicating shock or injury.

ARSENICUM ALBUM severe diarrhœa resulting from taking tainted food, and associated with vomiting, prostration, restlessness and anxiety. Stools are painless, scanty, brown in colour, excoriating to the skin and smelly. There is a desire for hot drinks.

BRYONIA profuse purging, coming on in the early morning and driving from bed; result of eating sour fruit or drinking cold water when over-heated.

CHAMOMILLA diarrhœa associated with teething in infants; slimy, grass-green stools which contain particles of undigested food, mucus and blood, and smell like bad eggs.

CHINA debilitating, painless diarrhœa with offensive stools; may result from a summer chill or from eating fruit.

COLOCYNTHIS frequent urging, severe colicky pains, somewhat relieved by pressure and bending double; stools are copious, thin, spluttery, frothy and saffron-yellow in colour. Sometimes the stools are small in bulk and there is temporary relief after the stool is passed.

DULCAMARA diarrhœa from getting cold and wet, or from sudden chilling when hot; stools slimy, green or yellow and may contain blood.

NUX VOMICA from dietary indiscretion, or diarrhœa alternates with constipation; WORSE in a.m. and after a big meal; much urging to stool; stools contain slime and blood; temporary relief after passage of stool.

PHOSPHORICUM ACIDUM painless diarrhœa, nervous in origin, or due to toxic state as in typhoid fever; profuse watery stools containing undigested food particles. Very definite relief is felt after passage of a stool.

PODOPHYLLUM urgent early morning painless diarrhœa, or diarrhœa preceded by severe colic; very profuse, spluttery, pea soup-like stools, passed in gushes and very offensive; WORSE after eating or drinking; passage of stool is followed by an empty, sinking feeling in the pit of the stomach.

PULSATILLA diarrhœa at night; diarrhœa from taking cold drinks, while eating, from nervousness, after eating onions, from rich food or pastry; very variable, no two stools alike.

SULPHUR diarrhœa drives the patient from bed in the early morning, about 5 a.m. The stools are painless and very variable in consistence and amount.

VERATRUM ALBUM is indicated when the acute diarrhœa is accompanied by vomiting and icy cold sweat. The patient wants iced water and wide open windows; may faint on the bathroom floor.

N.B.—Nervous diarrhœa will call for either ARGENTUM NITRICUM or GELSEMIUM (see pages 68 & 69).

Diphtheria—(see Sore Throat)

Dysentery

This term is used when stools are extremely frequent, accompanied by much pain and terrible urging, and contain little but blood and mucus. The large bowel is inflamed and the infection is either bacillary or amœbic. In an epidemic, or in districts where either type of the disease is common, precautions should be taken.

Nothing should be eaten in the raw state, all milk should be boiled, meals served hot, and scrupulous hygiene be observed, both personal and in the kitchen. Hands must be frequently washed and individual, not communal, towels used. Flies must be excluded from contact with food by every available means. Disinfectant must be used in toilets and latrines, and access of flies prevented as far as possible.

Some of the modern drugs are proving of value in these conditions. Homœopathic remedies corresponding to the symptom pictures are as follows and can be administered in the usual way (30 or 6, at shorter or longer intervals according to the severity of the symptoms and the measure of relief):

ACONITUM very acute onset in hot weather or in hot climate.

CANTHARIS shreddy, blood-stained stools, with appalling straining and burning, painful urination.

CAPSICUM symptoms accompanied by terrific thirst and by shivering when drinking; much straining, and burning sensation in rectum.

IPECACUANHA symptoms accompanied by severe nausea and vomiting; constant call to stool, cannot get off the pan; very slimy stools.

MERCURIUS CORROSIVUS perhaps the most important remedy in this disorder, symptoms very acute, stools hot, slimy, offensive and contain a great deal of blood; cutting pains in rectum and straining not relieved by passage of stool.

Earache

As mentioned in the section on accidents, ears must be treated with great respect, gentleness and caution. Earache is usually due to inflammation behind the ear drum, often conveyed from the throat along the Eustachian tube. Medical advice and aid should be sought as it might be advisable to incise a bulging ear drum to externalise the infection and prevent inward spread with mastoid involvement. As an immediate measure to counteract the pain in the ear one of the following remedies can be given (a few doses of 30 or 6):

ACONITUM acute onset, violent pain, some relief from local heat.

BELLADONNA digging, throbbing pain, often on right side; face red and hot. The pain is aggravated by the least jar. Heat gives relief. Thirst is not marked.

CHAMOMILLA pain made **WORSE** by local heat; child very cross and fretful, but may be *BETTER* if carried; pains very severe, extorting cries.

HEPAR SULPHURIS stitching pains, sore throat, desire to be warmly wrapped up, tenderness over mastoid process; peevish, nothing pleases. The condition is made **WORSE** by the least draught. It may start in the left ear and spread to the right.

PULSATILLA brought on by chilling when hot or after getting wet; may accompany an infectious fever; pain is **WORSE** from heat; child is weepy and wants attention and company.

A few drops of PLANTAGO mother tincture may be instilled into the painful ear.

Eye Affections

Any serious trouble in connection with the eyes must always receive the most expert care and attention without any delay. There are, however, some eye conditions to which reference can be made here with advantage.

Black specks before the eyes

It is not at all an uncommon experience to notice small black specks or twirligigs apparently floating in front of the eyes. Moreover they change position readily with every movement of the eyes or head. They seem more obvious some days and less noticeable at other times.

These specks and spirals rejoice in the name of *muscae volitantes,* and have been attributed to various causes without much confirmatory evidence. In any case they are of little significance and can be disregarded. If especially troublesome a few doses of AGARICUS, CHINA, NUX VOMICA, or PHOSPHORUS, 30 or 6, according to general indications, may afford relief.

Bloodshot eye

Inflammations of the eye, whether superficial or deep, are accompanied by redness, often of a dusky hue, as well as by pain and distress. These call for treatment by an eye specialist. But occasionally, often without obvious cause, a flaming patch of red discoloration may be observed to one or other side of the pupil and iris. This is due to a hæmorrhage beneath the conjunctiva and outside the actual eyeball. It is somewhat alarming in appearance but more unsightly than serious in significance.

A few doses of ARNICA 30 or 6 will speed recovery and allay any pain that may be present. If absorption of the blood is delayed LEDUM may be substituted for the ARNICA.

Eye strain

This is a rather vague term and usually refers to a sore, tired sensation in the eyes, attributed rightly or wrongly to over-use. It is, of course, necessary to check the vision for any error of refraction which may need correction by glasses. There may be occupational causes related to the type of work engaged in, or the lighting of the room in which the work is carried out; and it may be possible to make adjustments in respect of such causes of strain.

Remedies which may help in this condition (6 two or three times daily for a week or two, till relief is obtained) are as follows :

AGARICUS letters seem to swim or move when reading; twitching in lids; eyeballs oscillate from side to side; may see double.

CAUSTICUM vision dim; film before eyes; desire to close eyes; lids feel heavy; eye muscles weak.

GELSEMIUM vision dim; eyeballs sore, especially on moving them; eyelids droop, feel very heavy; possibly double vision.

JABORANDI (PILOCARPUS) eyes tire easily; sensation of heat and burning; indistinct vision; contracted pupils; white spots before eyes.

NATRUM MURIATICUM eyes give out while reading or sewing; letters or stitches "run together"; eyeballs feel too large; objects appear ringed with fiery zig-zags; hot tears stream down face when reading; lids feel gritty; spasmodic closure of lids.

PHOSPHORUS vision obscured by mist, or veil; red mist or black spots before eyes; eyes tire easily on use; sees better by shading eyes with hand.

RUTA weakness of vision with blurring; eyes ache while in use; eyes feel hot and burning, especially in evening; eyes water; green halo seen round artificial light; spasm of lower lids.

Lachrymation

A watery or other discharge from the eye calls for expert attention, especially if severe or persistent. As an immediate measure pending fuller investigation one or other of the following remedies may be given (a few doses of 30 or 6 till better):

ARSENICUM ALBUM much burning in eye; discharge which is hot and excoriating ; intense photophobia.

ALLIUM CEPA streaming eyes and nose, associated with much sneezing; discharge makes nose sore but not skin around eye.

EUPHRASIA eyes water all the time; discharge is burning and acrid; constant blinking.

PULSATILLA profuse yellow discharge, which does not excoriate the skin; WORSE in warm room; lids sore.

For bathing the eye either EUPHRASIA or HYPERICUM can be used as lotion (two drops of the mother tincture to the eye-bath of water).

Quivering Lids

Sometimes a sudden quivering or twitching is felt in one or other eyelid. This is a distressing sensation and seems to occur for no apparent reason. It usually passes off quite quickly and is not a cause for alarm. Various remedies are recommended in this condition, among them AGARICUS, BELLADONNA, CALCAREA CARB. and CICUTA (6 two or three times a day for a few days).

Styes

Recurrent styes on the eyelids will call for careful assessment on constitutional lines by a homœopathic physician. Various remedies may have to be considered but in many cases GRAPHITES, PULSATILLA or SULPHUR will give relief, 30 for a few doses or 6 twice a day for a longer period.

As a local application a compress of HYPERICUM lotion (ten drops of the mother tincture to the half pint of water) should be helpful.

Fever

The fact that the temperature of the body is raised above normal is usually an indication of increased activity on the part of the body's defence functions. This is frequently in response to infection of one kind or another and is a good sign as evidencing ability on the part of the individual to react.

A high temperature is, therefore, not in itself a symptom to be dealt with by drastic anti-pyretic (fever-reducing) drugs. Such treatment may indeed add to the strain on the body's vital functions and still further embarrass the heart and circulation. The fever will abate when the infection has been overcome or brought under control, and treatment should be aimed at assisting the body in its total task and not merely in relation to the one item of elevated temperature.

Apart from exceedingly high temperature of the range of 106—107 degrees F. which call for cold sponging, the treatment should be aimed at combatting infection, giving the body rest, and maintaining fluid balance. The best way to combat infection is to boost the body's own defences and this can be done effectually by the use of homœopathic remedies, but if a response is not rapid expert medical opinion will need to be sought, and this will equally be the case if the fever is accompanied by untoward signs or symptoms suggesting serious illness.

The following remedies have been found of value in febrile states, according to the indications present (30 repeated at four to eight hour intervals till better, or 6 three times daily):

ACONITUM skin dry and burning; face red but pale on sitting up; chills which pass from the extremities to the chest and head; intense thirst; great restlessness and agitation; fear of death; WORSE in evening and before midnight.

APIS absence of thirst; WORSE heat in any form; skin alternately dry and moist, but no heavy sweats; local patches of rosy swelling with burning and stinging sensation (red hot needles piercing flesh); frequent chills; possibly delirium or patient lies inert, face and eyes suffused, head rolled from side to side, body shaken at intervals by spasms, meningitic cry uttered in sleep.

ARSENICUM ALBUM excessively restless and agitated; anguish and fear of death; WORSE after midnight; prostration rapid and extreme; burning pains, but wants warmth (except to head); hot and cold alternately, and thirsty when hot for small amounts; possibly violent delirium with hallucinations.

BAPTISIA rapidly becomes gravely ill; temperature very irregular; highest at 11 a.m.; bruised battered sensation, as if in pieces all over the bed; dusky face, mentally confused, torpid, drops to sleep while replying to a question; tongue streaked down centre with white or brown. This remedy has proved of great value in both enteric and typhus fevers.

BELLADONNA high temperature; skin burning hot; face blazing red; pulse bounding; belligerent delirium; severe chills; general sweats; hallucinations; variable thirst.

BRYONIA shivery, sweating, thirsty for large amounts of cold water at long intervals; severe pains. WORSE least movement; face dusky red; tongue coated white; severe headache, WORSE by false step, moving head, or coughing; painful cough; delirium at night, lies with eyes closed, dwells on business affairs, asks to be taken home when in own bed all the time.

CHINA three-phase fever; chills and severe shaking give way to great heat, and this is followed by profuse sweating accompanied by intense thirst and prostration; bitter taste in mouth.

EUPATORIUM PERFOLIATUM useful in the "influenza type" of fever; temperature highest at 7 to 9 a.m.; severe chills; terrific thirst; muscles ache and bones feel as if they would break; sweats, but not during the chill.

FERRUM PHOSPHORICUM fever of rather indeterminate type; pulse rapid and full, but soft and compressible; moderate thirst; frequent sweats which afford no relief; shivery; red face; throbbing head; wants head cool.

GELSEMIUM absence of thirst; chills up and down spine; head feels hot and full; headache WORSE least movement, light or noise; wants to lie in dark and be quiet; torpor, trembling, possibly violent to the extent of wanting to be held down to stop the shaking; great heaviness of eyes and limbs.

IPECACUANHA a short chill accompanied by thirst; this is followed by heat all over except in the extremities which are icy cold and covered with clammy sweat; intense nausea, unrelieved by vomiting which causes great exhaustion; tongue clean.

MERCURIUS of special value at the onset of influenza-type fever associated with naso-pharyngeal symptoms; fever brought on by change to humid weather; creeping chills; chilliness alternates with burning heat; cold in patches; profuse sweats which give no relief; symptoms WORSE at night; breath foul, tongue flabby, pale, indented by teeth, and coated yellow; extreme thirst despite the moist mouth.

PHOSPHORUS fever and chills alternate; thirsty during hot spells, hungry during chills; sweats at night or in early hours, especially on head, hands and feet; chest involvement; delirium associated with exhaustion and apathy.

PYROGENIUM fevers of septic type, with swinging irregular temperature, and frequent chills and rigors; pulse weak and rapid, even when temperature falls; aches and pains all over; extreme restlessness despite the weakness; tongue dry, red, as if varnished; all secretions have a foul odour; coldness and pallor of surface.

RHUS TOXICODENDRON fever with great weakness and prostration, but nevertheless restless in the extreme; constantly turns and tosses in vain search for ease; mental confusion; tongue thickly coated, but red at tip; great thirst.

STRAMONIUM very high temperature; furious delirium; red face; staring eyes; terrible hallucinations; desire to escape; WORSE in dark, but cannot stand bright light.

Fibrositis

This term has for long been a favourite diagnosis label in ailments associated with sharp pains, aches in various parts of the body, especially, neck, back and limbs. Pains in the lower portion of the back have been called lumbago. A recent and popular diagnosis in many of these conditions is "slipped disc".

There are, of course, various tissues and structures in the regions affected which can suffer damage by strain or become inflamed as the result of irritation from without or from within (the body often manufactures its own poiscns or irritants, which cause inflammatory reactions in one or other of its tissues).

A disc, the fibrous pad or cushion between two adjacent vertebral bones, may on occasion become nipped or damaged, especially when a sudden movement is made without adequate guarding by supporting muscles; ligaments or muscle attachments may be wrenched or strained with resulting local swelling and involvement of nerves, causing pain. Or, as mentioned above, the same state of affairs may be brought about without any actual injury or trauma. In any case there are sharp pains owing to nerve involvement and usually local tenderness on pressure over the affected spots or area.

This condition may be brought about by physical stress, by exposure to inclement weather, by auto-intoxication or by some other elusive and ill-explained cause. The usual indication is for rest and warmth, possibly assisted by gentle massage and movement to avoid stiffness. Too energetic manipulation or too active movement may easily add further damage and make things worse. Remedies taken internally can be of great help and some of these are as follows (a few doses of 30, or more prolonged use of 6, till relief is obtained):

ACONITUM sudden onset of severe pains after exposure to dry cold winds; WORSE every movement, in warm room at night; thirsty, restless, touchy, scared.

APIS burning, stinging, stitching pains, whole back feels tired and bruised, WORSE heat and least movement; restless, irritable, depressed, wants to be uncovered and cool.

ARNICA spine very sensitive; spasms in muscles of neck and back; feels bruised, as if "bed too hard"; WORSE from mcvement but has to keep moving; morose, irritable.

BELLADONNA violent cutting or tearing pains, in neck, spine or hips; walks restlessly to and fro in search of ease; WORSE when at rest; blazing hot, bellicose, bed seems to be "surging up and down".

BERBERIS paralytic pain, shoulders, arms, hands, legs, feet, beneath nails; thighs feel cold; heels sore; WORSE walking; weakness and tiredness.

BRYONIA pains in nape, back, limbs; after exposure to dry cold, especially east winds; RELIEF from heat; WORSE least movement; anxious, ill-at-ease, peevish, great thirst for large amounts at long intervals.

CAUSTICUM drawing and tearing pains in limbs, especially at back of knee, with stiffness or weakness; lower limbs very restless at night; RELIEF in warm moist weather; WORSE cold winds. draughts and taking coffee.

CHAMOMILLA pains drive from bed at night to walk the floor; arms "go to sleep" when grasping objects; temper in a turmoil, nothing is right, pains are intolerable.

KALI BICHROMICUM wandering pains, felt especially in fingers and wrists; pain at bottom of spine when sitting; WORSE cold air, when snow is melting, 2 a.m. to 5 a.m.; cross and listless.

KALI CARBONICUM stitching cutting pains, often stabbing while at rest; pains extending up and down back and into thighs; WORSE walking; on attempting to walk feels as if "back would break"; firm pressure in small of back gives *RELIEF*; irritable, touchy, can't stand noise.

LEDUM pains which shift rapidly and spread centrally; associated with great stiffness; *RELIEF* from cold; WORSE heat, movement, after sitting still for a while, least pressure.

NUX VOMICA pains which come on after a wetting, or over-exertion, especially in lower part of back; hurts to turn in bed; muscles seem paralysed; cramps in calves or soles at night; WORSE dry cold, before rain, first thing in a.m.; *RELIEF* when rain actually falling, firm pressure, towards end of day.

PULSATILLA shooting pains in nape and elsewhere; neck and shoulders "crack" on movement; legs feel heavy in daytime and ache at night; WORSE heat, stuffy room, first movement, evening and first part of night; *RELIEF* from gentle movement and from pressure.

RHUS TOXICODENDRON one of the most useful remedies in this condition; pains brought on by over-exertion or exposure to cold and wet; back pain is relieved by bending body backwards; finger tips feel numb on grasping objects; pains and stiffness WORSE after rest, and *BETTER* by continued movement; extreme restlessness of mind and body.

Hay Fever

This most distressing and obstinate affliction, like asthma, presents a highly individual problem. The sufferer possesses a nose that is extraordinarily sensitive to changes in the composition of the air breathed.

Seasonal variations in the atmosphere, contamination of the air with dust, pollens, or some other irregular constituents will induce the violent reactions in the nose and eyes that are spoken of as hay fever. A more accurate term would be allergic rhinitis as hay is by no means the only offender. The fault lies in the individual and is a capacity for allergic (over-active) response to what are often unavoidable irritants in the air.

The problem of treatment is a knotty one; it can probably be handled best by the homœopathic approach because this takes into account the individual factors in the case. For adequate control, or cure, each case of hay fever presents a separate and distinct problem requiring skilled assessment along constitutional and miasmatic (toxicotic) lines. It is the deep-seated reactive capacity of the individual sufferer that has to be modified and rendered less vulnerable.

However in the matter of immediate relief of an actual attack certain remedies have been found of use, among them the following (two or three doses daily of 30 or 6 till better):

ALLIUM CEPA nose and eyes stream; sneezing is severe and of increasing frequency; lip and nostrils become sore; WORSE indoors, in morning, from contact with flowers and peach bloom.

ARSENICUM ALBUM sneezing violent and painful; violent tickle at one particular spot inside the nose, not relieved by sneezing; profuse watery discharge which burns the lip; WORSE change in weather; restless and worried.

ARUM TRIPHYLLUM sneezing is WORSE at night; much pricking in nose with desire to bore into nostril or pinch nose; nose is stuffed up, especially on left side, or runs profusely making nostril raw and sore; throat is also involved; eye symptoms are not severe.

DULCAMARA constant sneezing; nose stuffed up, or nose and eyes stream; eyes swell and water, then nose runs; then eyes water again; WORSE open air, damp, being chilled when hot, contact with newly cut hay.

EUPHRASIA much sneezing; discharge from nose is bland, but eye discharge is burning; throat often involved, with hard dry cough; WORSE open air, wind, lying down.

GELSEMIUM violent sneezing; nose streams in morning and discharge is excoriating; eyes feel hot and heavy ; much tingling in nose; throat dry and burning; swallowing causes pain in ears; face hot; aching all over, limbs feel heavy.

NUX VOMICA prolonged distressive spells of sneezing; nose apt to be stuffed up at night; excessive irritation in nose, eyes and face; itching extends to larynx and trachea; face feels as if close to a hot iron plate; chilly and irritable.

SABADILLA frequent spasms of severe sneezing; nose either stuffed up or running freely; much itching inside nose; eyelids red, face mottled; very sensitive to smell of flowers, fruit, garlic and other odours; extremely chilly; possibly associated with severe frontal headache or with bleeding from nose.

Headache

Headaches which persist, grow worse and incapacitate call for expert investigation. Headaches which recur at frequent intervals, are one-sided, and often accompanied by nausea and vomiting are known as migraine. These are of the nature of allergic reactions and are most hopefully handled by skilled individual assessment and treatment along homœopathic lines.

A great many "headache cures" are on the market, advertised, often enthusiastically, by their manufacturers and protagonists. Some of these are mere pain-killers; some contain drugs of dangerously toxic nature, which combine pain-relieving properties with risk to health or to life.

The homœopathic remedies capable of helping in the matter of headaches of one sort or another are many. In any particular case the choice of the simillimum may be extremely difficult. However as an immediate or emergency measure trial may be given to one of the following (a few doses of 30, or 6 for more prolonged use):

ACONITUM sudden violent headache; as if "skull contents would be forced out at the forehead"; as if "the skull were constricted by a ligature"; much throbbing in temples, first on one side, then on the other; restless, anxious, thirsty.

APIS stinging, stabbing, burning pain; occasional sharp cries; head bent backward or bored into pillow; feels bruised and tender all over; WORSE heat, warm room, hot bath; BETTER cold in every form; pain often occipital; patient alternately dry and hot or sweating.

ARGENTUM NITRICUM one-sided headache; pressive pain; head feels "much too large"; desire for cold air and cold drinks; WORSE mental effort, violent movement; BETTER tight bandage.

BELLADONNA bursting headache; violent throbbing, shooting; hot red face, dilated pupils; rush of blood to head; scalp very sensitive, pain comes on, also ceases, abruptly; WORSE least jar, movement, stooping, light, lying down; BETTER warm wraps to head, sitting upright, bending head backwards, firm pressure.

BRYONIA bursting, splitting, crushing headache; on attempting to sit up feels sick and faint; rush of blood to head, often with nose-bleed; drowsy, dry, peevish; hot flushed face; WORSE least movement or disturbance, hot room, coughing, straining at stool; BETTER lying quiet and motionless, firm pressure.

GELSEMIUM occipital headache associated with great heaviness of eyelids and limbs; vision blurred; hammering at base of brain; wants head high; feels exhausted, almost paralysed; WORSE mental effort, heat of sun, tobacco smoke; BETTER by passage of large quantities of pale urine; not thirsty.

GLONOINUM waves of terrible, bursting, throbbing pain, upward surges of hot blood; after-effect of exposure to hot sun; face purple or scarlet; WORSE heat, sun, every pulse beat, false step, least jar, weight of hat, bending head back; BETTER cool air or applications, lying down with head high, holding head in hands, after sleep.

NUX VOMICA splitting headache, or as if "a nail were driven into skull"; nausea and sour vomiting; wakes up with it, or comes on after eating; associated with stomach or liver complaints; after-effects of over-indulgence in food or alcohol; face red, hot, puffy; scalp sore to touch; WORSE open air, movement, mental effort; *BETTER* warmth, lying down, covering head, warm moist weather.

PULSATILLA periodic headache; pressive, distensive or throbbing; from eating ice-cream, rich food, or over-indulgence; feels nauseated and vomits sour food; head is hot and cool applications are desired; WORSE moving eyes, looking up, stooping, lying down; *BETTER* coolth, pressure, walking quietly in open air; weepy, craves air, not thirsty.

Heart Disease

The heart is a very remarkable and a very wise organ. It knows how to relax and, if beating at a reasonable rate, puts in a great deal of rest during the 24 hours. For each contraction of the heart muscle (systole) is followed by a rest period (diastole), while the heart fills up again.

It is the job of the heart to deliver an adequate amount of blood into the circulation; it is the job of the circulation to distribute and shunt the blood so that every cell and organ of the body may receive its proper supply of oxygen and nutriment, and extra supplies to meet immediate local needs in response to special activity or exertion.

Failure on the part of the circulation to supply sufficient blood to the heart muscle, as occurs in coronary disease, or failure to return an adequate quantity of blood to the heart, as occurs in "shock" will embarrass the heart and interfere with its function. Weakness of the heart muscle, leaky valves, irregular heart rhythm may also embarrass the circulation because insufficient blood is pumped into it. Obviously, therefore, the heart and the circulation are dependent on one another, and disease of either the heart itself or the blood-vessels will interfere with the all important function of tissue nutrition. Moreover the task of elimination, removal of waste or toxic products, via the lungs, the skin, the kidneys and the bowel, is also dependent on an adequate performance by heart and circulation.

Apart from congenital abnormalities the heart may suffer damage in its muscle, its valves, its blood-vessels, or in the nervous mechanism which controls the rhythm and rate of its action. Slight damage may cause little distress or interference with function. Moreover symptoms of pain, palpitation, or distress in the region of the heart, may be due to causes outside the heart altogether, "wind" for example, and may occur in the absence of any disease of the organ. Again a heart with a "murmur" or a heart which reacts violently to psychological stress, may be a perfectly efficient one.

The important thing is the test of performance. A somewhat damaged heart can often carry out its task quite efficiently provided that it is protected from overstrain by the sensible avoidance of stress, both physical and emotional, on the part of its owner. A life of invalidism is usually not called for but merely a wise restriction of activity within reasonable limits, varying with the individual.

The presence of symptoms suggestive of disorder of the heart calls for careful investigation as to cause. This will often include X-rays and an electro-cardiographic test. The treatment of heart disease must, therefore, be under the direction of a doctor, and homœopathy has many remedies of proven value.

Herpes Labialis

This affection, commonly spoken of as "cold sore", is a frequent accompaniment of colds or infective conditions such as pneumonia. A cluster of small vesicles or blebs appear on the lips or nostrils, possibly preceded by a sensation of heat or burning. The eruption should be left severely alone and will dry up in the course of five to ten days. Its disappearance may be encouraged and the recurrence of fresh eruptions discouraged by the use of NATRUM MUR. or RHUS TOX. (a few doses of 30 or 6).

Herpes Zoster

The common name for this complaint is "shingles". It is ascribed to a virus identical with that responsible for or, at any rate, associated with chicken-pox. The tissues mainly involved are the roots of a spinal or cranial nerve, and an eruption of little blisters on a red base appears along the line of distribution of the nerve affected. This may be on the trunk or head, or indeed anywhere on the body. The appearance of the rash is preceded by very severe neuralgic pain and general malaise. The latter usually clears up when the rash appears, but the pain sometimes is more persistent.

The ordinary treatment of this most distressing complaint is none too satisfactory, as evidenced by the large number of drugs listed for its palliation. Homœopathic remedies of proven worth in allaying pain and aiding recovery (a few doses of 30, or 6 for a longer period) are:

APIS large blebs, much swelling, part affected burns and stings and cool applications afford relief.

ARSENICUM ALBUM confluent eruption, severe burning pain, great restlessness and anxiety, sleepless after midnight.

MEZEREUM very severe pain and itching; scratching causes burning sensation; brown scabs form.

RANUNCULUS BULBOSUS severe burning pain with much itching; WORSE touch, movement, taking food.

Hiccough

This curious and unpleasant affliction is due to a sudden involuntary jerky contraction of the diaphragm associated with a simultaneous closure of the glottis. The spasm of the diaphragm produces an inspiration and the approximation of the vocal cords interrupts the incoming stream of air with the resultant "hic" sound.

An attack of hiccoughs may appear out of the blue for no apparent reason. In many instances there is some form of irritation at the lower end of the gullet which fires off the reflex. At other times the cause is deeper, in the nervous system or associated with a toxic state. Usually an attack is short-lived but sometimes the spasms may persist and prove obdurate, and cause great distress and exhaustion.

Hiccough in infants can usually be relieved by feeding a little water or milk. In older subjects a variety of manœuvres are recommended as possibly efficacious in cutting short the attack. Hippocrates suggested a pinch of snuff to induce sneezing. Simple dodges often employed are: holding the breath as long as possible; breathing rapidly and deeply; breathing in and out of a paper bag; drinking cold water while holding the breath; and pulling the tongue forward. In severe cases other medical measures may have to be used, and possible causes investigated.

Remedies which may be used homœopathically (a few doses of 30, at intervals of a quarter to half an hour apart) are :

ARSENICUM ALBUM attack brought on by taking cold drinks, or during fevers, at the time when the temperature is expected to rise.

CAJUPUTI obstinate attacks on slightest provocation, such as laughing, talking or taking food: (one or two drops of the oil on sugar; or 3rd potency).

CICUTA attacks violent and noisy, possibly associated with convulsions.

HYOSCYAMUS onset after eating; possibly associated with convulsions; attack occurring at night; post-operative hiccough.

IGNATIA attack brought on by eating, by smoking, or by emotional upset.

MAGNESIUM PHOSPHORICUM very obstinate type, associated with persistent soreness.

NICCOLUM very severe attack associated with thirst; may come on in evening.

NUX VOMICA attack associated with digestive disturbance; may follow indiscretion in diet, either solid or liquid.

PULSATILLA attack caused by taking cold drinks or by tobacco smoke.

RANUNCULUS BULBOSUS hiccough associated with alcoholism.

STRAMONIUM follows taking hot drinks, violent.

TABACUM attack brought on by coughing.

VERATRUM ALBUM attack follows taking hot drinks or after a bout of vomiting.

Indigestion

This term denotes disorder in the digestive functions sufficient to cause discomfort. It may be temporary or persistent. The distress may be slight or severe. When symptoms of digestive disorder appear in an individual previously quite free from such complaints, and are either severe or persistent, adequate investigation as to possible causes must be carried out.

Indigestion may be the result of faulty habits of eating or drinking, dietary indiscretion, either episodic or habitual. This is obvious but what is less obvious, and often not sufficiently realised, is that indigestion may also be the result of faulty habits of thought.

Mental tension, inadequately countered by a healthy nonchalance and proper periods of leisure and relaxation; fear and anxiety; rage and resentment; impatience and irritation; these and allied harmful emotions are potent disturbers of digestive rhythm and well-being.

These mischievous tensions cause indigestion in three ways. They interfere with the tone of the muscle in the wall of the stomach and gut, which leads to spasm or over-distension. Also the normal rhythm of the bowel movements is upset. Both these deviations from the normal result in discomfort, disorder or pain. But in addition the tone of the muscle in the walls of the blood vessels is affected, and localised vaso-spasm may seriously embarrass the circulation so vital to the proper function and health of the digestive organs. Finally there is interference with the timely secretion and flow of the juices essential to adequate digestion of food.

As the outcome of these interferences with normal function not only may much distress and pain be experienced but actual tissue damage may occur causing so-called "organic" disease. Thus the necessity for avoidance of unwholesome food is paralleled by an even greater need for avoidance of emotional upset and mental stress. The one error "throws a spanner into the digestive works", which is bad enough, but the other upsets the control of the whole digestive function at the centre and this may be even worse in its long-term harmful effects.

A term much bandied about in connection with indigestion is "acidity". The contents of the stomach are, of course, acid in reaction. It is only when, instead of going on downwards, there is a back-flow into the gullet, or even into the throat, that the sensation of heartburn and the awareness of acidity is experienced. This may be countered with an alkali such as sodium bicarbonate or one of the hundreds of anti-acid medicaments on the market, but as soon as the acid is neutralised and the stomach contents become alkaline, a fresh flow of acid secretion is called forth. The relief is, therefore, only temporary.

Various remedies have been found helpful when used homœopathically in connection with digestive disorders. Among them (30 for a few doses, or 6 for longer periods) are :

ANACARDIUM heartburn; pain and fullness in pit of stomach 2 to 3 hours after food; foul breath, bad taste in mouth; hollow sinking feeling, or "plug" sensation in belly; WORSE cold drinks, heat of sun, emotional stress; *BETTER* taking food, especially warm food, and by onward passage of flatus.

ARSENICUM ALBUM burning pain in pit of stomach quite soon after food, or shortly after midnight; sensation of weight like a stone in stomach; painful retching and vomiting leading to great exhaustion with icy coldness; constant thirst for small amounts; WORSE least quantity food, cold drinks, pressure on pit of stomach; *BETTER* warmth, warm drinks, after vomiting.

BRYONIA distress in stomach pit soon after food, with heaviness "like a stone"; nausea and faintness on attempting to sit up; waterbrash; biliousness; dull pain in liver region; heartburn; hiccough; thirst for large quantities but warm drinks are vomited; WORSE chill, pressure, vinegar, oysters; *BETTER* lying quite still on back, and, to some extent, by belching.

CARBO VEGETABILIS pain and tenderness in pit of stomach about half an hour after food, with spread to chest, back and along spine; heaviness, waterbrash, much bloating; offensive flatus; aversion from meat, milk, fat; desire for sweet things and salty foods; internal heat with external coldness, and great desire for air; WORSE even simplest food, ice-cream; *BETTER* sitting up and, temporarily, by belching.

GRAPHITES constrictive pain in pit of stomach about 2 hours after food; "lump in throat" with constant desire to retch or swallow; dribbles saliva during sleep; eructations taste of food or acid; feels nauseated, weak and trembly in a.m.; may vomit after food; much burning, griping and bloating; aversion from meat, fish, salt, sweets; salty taste or burning blisters in mouth; irritable, fidgety; *BETTER* eating food, drinking hot fluids, especially milk, lying down, belching, passing wind.

HEPAR SULPHURIS burning, heaviness, pressure in stomach pit, even after small meal; severe bloating; frequent belching; faintness in mid-morning; bilious attacks; sticking pain in liver region; desire for vinegar, wine, spicy food; aversion from fat; talks fast, drinks rapidly; very peevish; WORSE when walking; *BETTER* after eating.

HYDRASTIS constant pain in pit of stomach, as from a hard-cornered object; feels horribly ill, nothing tastes right, vomits everything taken, loathing for food; bitter taste in mouth, tongue feels burnt; WORSE bread and vegetables especially.

KALI BICHROMICUM heartburn and "weight" immediately after food, with pain which spreads to back between shoulder-blades; may be small spot of soreness and tenderness below ribs on left side; possibly a hunger pain about 3 hours after food; this is *BETTER* after taking food; nausea and lack of appetite in morning; vomiting of sour fluid, stringy mucus, bile; aversion from water; desire for beer and acids; intolerance for meat; mouth dry, tongue glazed or yellow, indented by teeth; listless with great desire to lie down.

NUX VOMICA heartburn, cramping, clawing, throbbing pain and great feeling of weight, 1 to 2 hours after food; severe bloating several hours after eating; waterbrash, hawking, retching, ineffectual inclination to vomit; pain spreads to back between the shoulder-blades and to the chest; queasy nausea in a.m.; pit of stomach very sensitive; desire for fat, beer, brandy; aversion from meat, coffee, water, tobacco; WORSE lack of exercise, loss of sleep, alcohol, coffee, tobacco; *BETTER* hot food and fluids, after stool.

PULSATILLA much bloating, sensation as if "had eaten too much" or "a stone in stomach", 1 to 2 hours after food; food regurgitates; eructations taste of food; raw, scraped sensation in throat and burning in stomach; foul taste in mouth in morning; vomiting of food taken some hours previously, especially after emotional stress; odd cravings for indigestible things or some special food or drink, e.g. herrings, lemon drink; absence of thirst; WORSE warm room, warm food, rich food, in evening after supper; *BETTER* temporarily from taking cold things.

Influenza

"The flu" is a convenient term commonly employed in connection with certain types of infectious illness, occurring at times in epidemic form. The onset is usually sudden and the illness is often rendered more severe by unwise attempts to "keep going" and "carry on". Various causal agents have been described in the past; at the present time the infective organism is said to be a virus of "great complexity and diversity".

Fortunately a number of remedies used in the homœopathic manner are available to afford relief and hasten cure, among these are the following (a few doses of 30 at four hourly intervals, or 6 for a longer period):

ARSENICUM ALBUM streaming eyes and nose, chilliness and very great prostration.

BAPTISIA very rapid prostration, high fever, gastric symptoms, stuporous state, looks drugged, with dull red face, complains of feeling "all in bits".

BRYONIA very hot, very dry, wants to lie quite still and be let alone; aches all over and headache is **WORSE** least movement and *BETTER* pressure; chest symptoms; tongue is coated white; great thirst for cold fluids; cough causes headache; irritable and, if delirious, talks of business or "wants to go home" when at home.

EUPATORIUM PERFOLIATUM very severe pains in limbs and back, bones feel "broken", dare not move for pain; bursting headache; shivering, and chills in back; chill begins at 7 to 9 a.m.; eyeballs sore.

GELSEMIUM chills run up and down spine, cold and hot alternately, great heaviness and tiredness of body and limbs, and especially head and eyelids; aches and pains all over; sneezing; hard cough; absence of thirst; bursting headache from behind forward to eyes and forehead; relief from passing large quantities of pale urine.

NUX VOMICA intractably chilly, cold even in bed, and least movement or exposure intensifies the sensation of cold; fresh shivering and chill after drinking; aching in limbs and back; stomach upset; nose stuffed up at night.

PYROGENIUM severe pains in back and thighs; chilliness no fire can warm; creeping chills in back with thumping heart; very rapid pulse with temperature not proportionately high; intense restlessness; violent pulsations; bursting headache; bed feels "too hard"; feels beaten, bruised all over.

For prevention in the case of contacts GELSEMIUM 30 may be given, three doses spread over a 24 hour period, or three doses of the remedy that is being found to be effective in any current epidemic.

Insomnia

There have been many theories put forward to explain the physiology of sleep. It seems probable that during waking hours a multitude of stimuli due to muscular and mental activity, the impact of light, noise, and the environment generally, ensure wakefulness and prevent sleep. When these stimuli are cut off, or cut down by lying still, relaxing muscles, shutting out light and noise to a great extent, and ceasing mental activity sleep is the natural outcome.

There are, of course, plenty of nervous impulses reaching the brain from within the body even when the outside stimuli are cut down. Some of these are physical due to bowel movements, alterations in the circulation, distension of the urinary bladder, various disorders capable of causing distress or pain and so on. Some are psychological due to emotional tension, mental activity, or subconscious thought processes. It is often this type of stimulus that interferes with sleep despite the cutting down of the more obvious external and physical stimuli.

Natural sleep is to be wooed with all earnestness and persistence as the alternative, drug-induced sleep, carries with it a host of undesirable possibilities, not the least the danger of drug-addiction. It is of great importance to cultivate the art of not taking problems to bed with one, of laying one's head on the pillow and drifting off into nowhere, with both mind and body fully relaxed.

If thoughts, anxious or even pleasant, crowd and persist an act of will is required to switch on to a separate line of thought altogether and keep on it, deliberately refusing to follow the line of thought that distresses or disturbs and thus prevents sleep. Persistence in this manœuvre will result in the ability not only to "think of something else" but to think of nothing at all, the prelude to dropping off to sleep and staying asleep. If awakened by some internal or environmental stimulus, possibly a vivid dream or sudden noise, the same manœuvre can be repeated.

The notion that one must have at least so many hours sleep per night is, of course, fallacious. In habit of sleep and in sleep requirements people vary greatly, as in so many other ways. Alarm over apparent lack of sleep merely serves to increase nervous tension and make sleep the more elusive. Calm and confidence have the opposite effect. Each must discover for himself, or herself, the habits of diet, exercise, relaxation and mental occupation that are most conducive to a good night's sleep.

The benefit of homœopathic treatment on general health often includes an improvement in sleeping habit. A number of remedies have also been found of use in this connection though their employment without attention to the general principles mentioned above is likely to prove disappointing. Some of these are listed below (a 6 taken half an hour or so before bedtime and repeated on getting into bed, a 30 perhaps nightly for a few nights, or even a 200 in the event of great stress or strain, but not repeated more than once or twice):

ACONITUM kept awake by sensation of fear or panic, insomnia after shock or fright; restless tossing.

ARNICA sleep prevented by over-tiredness, either physical or mental; bed feels too hard; must keep moving in search of relief.

ARSENICUM ALBUM sleepless after midnight from anxiety and restlessness; has to get up and walk the floor.

BELLADONNA sleepy yet unable to sleep; child tosses, kicks clothes off, twitches; restless sleep with frightful dreams; jerks awake when dropping off; surface heat.

CHAMOMILLA sleepless and restless, especially in first part of night; gets up and walks the floor; as soon as bedtime comes is wide awake; irritable and, if a child, wants to be carried all the time.

COFFEA utterly wide awake, mind active, possibly with pleasurable thoughts; result of sudden news, either exciting or distressing.

NUX VOMICA sleepless after mental strain or over-indulgence; wakes about 3 to 4 a.m. and after a wakeful period drops off, only to wake later cross, tired and unrefreshed; sleep dreamy and restless.

OPIUM feels sleepy but cannot get off; very acute hearing both near and far; clocks striking at a distance keep from sleep; bed feels hot, moves about in vain to find a cool spot.

PULSATILLA first sleep restless, and sound sleep when it is time to rise; gets too hot in bed, throws off covers, gets chilly and pulls them on again; put arms above head when asleep.

These remedies are mentioned for what they are worth, but as always with homœopathy the real problem is to study the individual and so correct disordered health as to restore normality, sleep included.

Lactation

The following remedies have proved of value in troubles connected with the breast-feeding of infants (a few doses of 30, or 6 for a longer period if so required):

BELLADONNA flow of milk too free; breasts inflamed, red, hot, swollen, tender, possibly stony hard; face flushed, skin hot and dry.

CALCAREA CARBONICA copious flow of watery milk, refused by infant; or milk scanty with distended breasts; patient is chilly, very averse cold air, pale, flabby, weak, apt to perspire, especially on head at night.

LAC DEFLORATUM diminished secretion of milk, decrease in size of breasts; feels very depressed and despondent; very thirsty.

PHYTOLACCA flow of milk is excessive; nipples extremely sore and nursing is very painful; pain radiates all over the body; breast hard, lumpy; possibly actual formation of pus.

PULSATILLA milk too scanty; nursing is painful and pains extend to chest, neck, back; or continued secretion of milk after weaning and breasts feel stretched, tense, sore; patient is mild and tearful, averse from stuffy heat and desiring plenty of cool air.

SILICEA milk suppressed; sharp pain in breasts; pain in back; increase in lochia; discharge of blood from nipple when attempts to nurse infant; child refuses milk or vomits after feed; breasts inflamed, deep-red in centre, rose-coloured elsewhere, hard, sensitive to touch; constant burning pain and high temperature.

Measles

This infectious fever, also known as Morbilli, should be avoided if possible. Not only is the original attack liable to be severe but there may be undesirable complications and aftermaths. To this end "contacts" should be given PULSATILLA 30, three doses during a 24 hour period, as a preventive measure.

During an attack of measles homœopathic treatment will aid recovery, diminish distress, and also discourage complications. In the early stages ACONITUM, BELLADONNA or FERRUM PHOSPHORICUM may be given according to the indications (see section on Fever). Other remedies which may be called for (30 for two or three days at 6 to 8 hourly intervals, or 6 three or four times daily for a few days) are:

APIS high temperature, very hot and wanting covers off; eyes sore; possibly ears involved; child tearful and irritable.

BRYONIA very tiresome cough on account of chest involvement; high temperature, dull look with swollen face; complains of headache; mouth dry with intense thirst for cold water; feels chilly, but wants air.

EUPHRASIA streaming nose and eyes, and latter sore with marked photophobia; moderate type of fever and does not feel very ill.

GELSEMIUM very high fever; delirium; extreme prostration; very dry tongue; possibly convulsions.

PHOSPHORUS chest symptoms marked; troublesome dry cough and feeling of tightness in chest; great thirst for cold water, which may be vomited when it warms in the stomach.

PULSATILLA very restless, very irritable; wants to be petted and constantly waited on; troublesome cough; desire for cool air.

Measles, German

This traditionally innocuous ailment, also known as Rubella, has in recent years been shown to have one serious significance. If acquired during pregnancy, especially during the first four months, it may have an adverse effect. For this reason, in the event of exposure to infection during pregnancy, or with a pregnancy in prospect, it would be wise to prescribe the RUBELLA NOSODE 30, (three doses during a 24 hour period).

Obviously also it is an advantage if the disease is contracted in early years and a natural immunity acquired in this way. At this age, therefore, the acquisition of the disease should be encouraged rather than prevented. If treatment is called for in an attack this should be along the lines described under the section on Fever.

Mouth Ulcers

There is sometimes a tendency for recurrent attacks of ulceration in the mouth causing considerable distress. It is important to pay attention to the general health. There are several remedies which may be of value :

BORAX is often effective with small ulcers of the aphthous type. The mouth is hot and tender; the ulcers tend to bleed if touched or when eating. There may be a mouldy taste in the mouth.

MERCURIUS is indicated when there is excessive salivation, spongy gums which bleed easily, a sweetish metallic taste in the mouth and marked thirst despite the fact that the mouth is quite moist.

NATRUM SULPHURICUM when there are small blisters or extremely sensitive ulcers, with relief from holding cold fluids in the mouth.

NITRICUM ACIDUM is called for when the ulcers are accompanied by sharp splinter-like pains, much salivation and fœtor oris.

Mumps

Prevention should be attempted by the administration to contacts of PAROTIDINUM or RHUS TOX 30. (three doses during a 24 hour period). In the treatment of mumps PILOCARPINUM MURIATICUM 3x is recommended by Burnett, and the effectiveness of this remedy is confirmed by Tyler. ACONITUM or BELLADONNA may be indicated by typical symptoms, or, at a later stage PULSATILLA. These will be given in the usual way (30 for a few days, three times a day, or 6 for perhaps a longer period). The patient should be confined to bed to diminish the risk of complications.

"Nerves"

It is quite common for a patient to be told he is suffering from "nerves"; and associated advice is often to "pull yourself together". Such advice is entirely mistaken for the patient whose "nerves" are a bit ragged or jittery is usually suffering from mental fatigue and emotional tension. The process of pulling oneself together, whatever that means, certainly would involve both effort and strain thus increasing the fatigue and adding to the tension.

Exactly the reverse is what is needed, namely a lazy and leisured recuperation of mental vigour and a nonchalant carefree relaxation of "taut nerves".

This may not be easy, and will be impossible if there is persistence in giving way to, or harbouring, the harmful type of emotion, which saps nervous energy and produces both psychological and physical tension.

The types of emotion that are hostile to health can be summed up as fear, fury and frustration. Fear includes such satellites as worry, anxiety and apprehension. Fury comprises anger, inward rage, brooding over wrongs (real or imagined), bottling things up, resentment, "the injured feeling" (closely akin to self-pity, a most harmful, unnecessary and unwise indulgence). Frustration finds expression in impatience, irritation, intolerance of persons or circumstances.

All such emotions, if persisted in, tend to produce tension and disturbance not merely of mind but also of various physical functions associated with secretion, circulation, digestion and so on. Per contra a consistent attitude of carefree cheerfulness, confidence and contentment is conducive to both peace of mind and ease of body.

This may appear to be a somewhat Utopian aim in this age of hectic hurry but it is not impossible of achievement, especially if every circumstance of environment and experience is regarded in the light of opportunity. The tendency to relate one's circumstances to oneself, as things that oppress, annoy, are unbearable, not to be tolerated and so on, must be resisted. Instead one must relate oneself to one's circumstances and go to meet them with quiet assurance, even with zest. It is the direction that matters.

No longer do circumstances hem one in and get one down, but they provide constant opportunity for endurance, for enjoyment, for interest, for entertainment, for achievement, for service. Life is no longer frustration; it is fun.

An established condition of nervous fatigue and emotional disturbance demands the care and guidance of a physician. A recourse to sedative drugs is not the answer. These tend to further depress the already depressed, and to interfere with that clarity of thought and reason so essential to the process of re-orientation. The issues are often quite simple if faced honestly and squarely, and not confused by a jumble of unintelligible jargon based on unsubstantiated hypotheses.

In times of sudden sorrow, stress, shock, and emotional upset from one cause or another a number of remedies have proved their worth (a dose or two of 200, a few doses of 30, or 6 for a short period):

ACONITUM acute anxiety; extreme impatience; horrible fears; intolerance of pain, music, least noise; confusion of mind; thoughts and ideas chase one another.

ARGENTUM NITRICUM fearful and apprehensive before ordeal of any kind; fear of heights, of crowds, of closed spaces, of water; stage fright; exam funk.

CAUSTICUM effects of grief or worry; unhappy, inclined to tears, hopeless; full of forebodings and vague fears; jumps at least noise; peevish, critical of others, forgetful.

CHAMOMILLA temper in a turmoil; everything wrong; extreme restlessness; trifles annoy; nothing pleases, everything intolerable.

GELSEMIUM depression, possibly after influenza; mind seems paralysed; listless, indolent, disinclined for any effort; fear of falling; apprehension before ordeal; tremulous and shaky.

IGNATIA effects of sudden shock or stress; depressed and irritable; moods alternate; bottles things up; dwells on sorrows in secret; cannot forget; involuntary tears; frequent sighing; goes to pieces when crossed; cannot bear pain.

KALI PHOSPHORICUM effects of prolonged strain; lassitude and depression; averse from meeting people; jumpy and starts at least thing; everything too much trouble.

NUX VOMICA chilly, tense, active person; constantly "frustrated"; quarrelsome, critical, hypersensitive, unduly exasperated by trifles; wants to throw things about.

PULSATILLA effects of bad news, anxiety, emotional upset, in mild, "touchy", weepy, type of person, fond of company and averse from solitude; upsets felt mainly in stomach and may cause vomiting.

Nettle-rash

This affliction, which also goes by the names hives and urticaria, is apt to occur in hypersensitive or allergic persons. It calls for expert medical attention but as an emergency measure and in the presence of sudden severe swellings which itch and burn, a few doses of APIS or URTICA URENS 30 or 6 may be given to obtain relief.

Obesity

Increase in weight is the common experience of those who are constitutionally prone to stoutness. Drastic slimming, especially by the use of drugs which interfere with normal physiological function, is prejudicial to health. On the other hand excessive weight should be controlled and this is largely a matter of attention to diet and fluid intake.

Volumes have been written and fortunes made, in relation to a great variety of dietary fads and régimes. Many of these are contradictory and the more one reads the greater the confusion, and "the less there is left to live upon". The fallacy of rigid régimes is that they omit to take into account the individual factor. That which suits one person may be quite unsuitable, or even harmful for another.

Pathological obesity may be the result of disease or may be induced by taking drugs, and will require expert investigation and guidance. But simple weight reduction is in the hands of the individual. The answer is to eat less and drink less, for fluids are retained in the body as weight. The following list of foods forbidden and foods allowed may serve as a useful guide, and avoid the time-consuming methods of weighing out dishes and "counting calories".

FOODS FORBIDDEN :

        duck, pork, fat meat, sausages:
        cakes, biscuits, buns, pastries :
        vermicelli, macaroni, all cereals :
        chocolate, cocoa :
        milk puddings, steamed puddings :
        sugar, jams :
        ice cream, cream, synthetic cream :
        sweetened, or evaporated, tinned milk :
        pulses, baked beans :
        thick soups, sauces, gravies, fried foods :
        grapes, bananas, tinned, dried or crystalised fruits :
        nuts, coconut :
        fruit cordials and squashes :
        beer, wines, cider, ginger ale.

FOODS ALLOWED :

        lean meat, except pork or duck :
        chicken, rabbit, tripe, sweetbreads :
        heart, liver, kidney :
        clear soups, meat extracts made with water :
        cheese, eggs (not scrambled or fried) :
        white fish, herring :
        all green vegetables, salads without dressing or oil,
            tomato, turnip, parsnip :
        fresh peas, runner beans :
        fruit served without sugar :
        milk, about $\frac{1}{2}$ pint daily :
        butter and margarine in restricted amounts :
        bread (whole meal) in restricted amounts :
        bran (bought at corn chandler's), if constipated, with
            all meals, about two tablespoonfuls per meal :
        potatoes in moderation.

Keep salt down to a minimum.
Limit fluid intake, all fluids included, to $2\frac{1}{2}$ or 3 pints daily.
Plenty of deep breathing and exercise.

Pain

Pain has protective value. It is nature's red light, a warning that things may be not as they should be in the body. Moreover pain in its location, character and type may be not only a warning but a guide to what is going wrong and an aid to the physician in diagnosis.

For these reasons the mere dulling of pain with drugs may be most unwise. To remove the appreciation of pain without correcting the cause, and by so doing perhaps obscure the cause, is obviously a procedure that is both futile and dangerous.

A warning must, therefore, be sounded against the ready resort to and indiscriminate use of pain-killers. Not only may these drugs interfere with accurate diagnosis and thus cause delay in adequate treatment, but many (if not most) of them are habit-forming and give rise to addiction.

A further warning must be given in connection with pain, namely that its absence does not necessarily mean that no serious disease is present in the body. Appreciation of the sensation of pain depends on adequate nerve-supply to the affected part and on proper nerve-impulse conduction. Some parts of the body are poorly supplied with nerve-endings; some disease processes interfere with nerve-conduction. When, therefore, there is some deviation from normal health or some unusual development in the body this should always call for expert medical investigation and attention *even though no pain may be present,* and such investigation should not be delayed.

Again when severe pain is present and there is sudden relief this may not mean that all is well and that the need for expert advice and care has passed. Indeed the reverse may be the case as in some acute abdominal conditions where the bursting of an inflamed organ under tension may give relief from pain but initiate an even more serious and urgent state of affairs than before. A really bad pain demands enquiry into the cause even after it has passed off, and the sooner the better, especially if other signs of disorder persist.

It is, of course, possible to have a lot of pain with only very slight cause, and it is also the case that the threshold of pain-awareness varies a great deal from one individual to another. The presence of pain should, therefore, be an occasion for alertness rather than necessarily for alarm. The first requisite is investigation as to the possible cause of the pain and only after this has been carried out should the question of pain-dulling drugs be considered.

Use of sedative or narcotic drugs carries disadvantages with the dual tendency to depression and drug addiction as a possible outcome. If relief can be obtained by drugs assisting natural curative processes so much the better. In this respect many of the remedies in the homœopathic materia medica have a reputation of proven worth (q.v. sectional references for different types of pain).

"Periods" and "Change of Life"

Disorders of the menstrual function, if serious or persistent, call for expert investigation and treatment. It is unwise to have recourse to pain-killing or other proprietary drugs as an alternative.

In connection with *amenorrhœa,* or suppression of the periods, the following remedies may be of value, i.e. in recent cessation of previously normal periods (a dose of 6 night and morning):

ACONITUM suppression following exposure to dry cold winds, or resulting from fright or shock.

BRYONIA suppression associated with vicarious menstruation, that is, bleeding from other sites such as the nose or the intestinal tract.

DULCAMARA suppression following a soaking or getting suddenly chilled when over-heated.

PULSATILLA suppression following getting the feet wet, or accompanied by nervous debility or by anæmia in the "pulsatilla" type of individual—pleasant, inclined to portliness, given to easy tears, averse from stuffy heat, wanting air, fond of rich food but upset thereby.

When there is much *pain with the period* the following remedies deserve mention (a dose of 6 every quarter or half hour till relief is obtained):

BELLADONNA cramping pains; early period with abundant flow of bright red blood; pains similar to pangs of child-birth and associated with pressure in the pelvis as if the contents would be expelled.

GELSEMIUM periods late and scanty; pains accompanied by sensation of great weight in the womb or as if the organ were being squeezed or crushed; pain extends to back or hips.

MAGNESIA PHOSPHORICA periods are early; shreds of membrane are mixed with blood; pains are neuralgic, severe, and somewhat relieved by bending double, by pressure, by heat applied locally.

NUX VOMICA in the 'nux' type of individual—lean, tense, irritable, excessively chilly, extremely active, loathing wind.

VIBURNUM OPULUS (this remedy is usually given in 3x potency in doses of five drops in a little water, three or four times a day) periods often delayed; severe cramping or bearing down pains, which extend to the thighs.

It is customary to attribute a variety of ills and distress to the "change of life" or menopause. This is probably both unnecessary and inaccurate inasmuch as the cessation of the monthly periods in the fourth or fifth decades is a normal physiological process. Further it would seem unwise to tamper with the body's own normal adjustment of its hormone balance by prescribing hormone preparations by mouth. Various remedies have been found helpful at this time of physiological adjustment. They should be prescribed under the guidance of a homœopathic physician with due regard to the individual indications in each case.

Piles or Haemorrhoids

This is a fairly common condition and may cause considerable pain and distress. There is a tendency to ascribe any bleeding or discomfort in the region of the rectum and anus to "piles". This is a very dangerous error as the cause of the bleeding or discomfort may be due to several other conditions, some serious and calling for skilled medical care.

It is, therefore, imperative that no diagnosis of piles should be assumed without careful expert examination, if necessary with the aid of proctoscope or sigmoidoscope.

Piles, if present, are clusters of enlarged varicose veins at the termination of the rectum. They are often the result of prolonged straining at stool on account of constipation, though there are other causes.

At first the piles, usually three in number, are soft and bleed readily. As time goes on they become larger and also more solid as the result of fibrosis, and tend to come down when a stool is passed. At first it is possible to replace the piles within the anal sphincter muscle, but in the long run they are liable to become permanently prolapsed, refusing to remain within the anus after replacement.

It may be advisable when this state of affairs has been reached to resort to surgical removal, which can give permanent relief. However, in the earlier stages homœopathic treatment can be of considerable benefit, once the diagnosis has been unequivocally confirmed.

A number of remedies claim attention. ALOE, HAMAMELIS, NITRICUM ACIDUM when there is bleeding and much soreness. If there is a tendency to prolapse then AESCULUS, LEDUM or PODOPHYLLUM should be considered. If there is severe pain and the piles are extremely sensitive to touch, PAEONIA, SILICEA or STAPHISAGRIA may be called for.

For external application PAEONIA ointment will often give relief. Attention to bowel movement and general health is necessary, and avoidance of alcohol. Any rectal complaint which proves unreponsive to treatment calls for expert investigation and advice.

Poliomyelitis

This infectious disease, involving especially the tissues of the central nervous system, presents a case for the most skilled and knowledgeable medical care. The risks associated with the condition, both immediate and remote, depend on which portion of the spinal cord is affected and also on the availability of adequate remedial aids. Opinion is still divided as to the best measures to be adopted in prevention, but the following precautions are advised to be taken by parents and children should the disease appear in their district :

Do not share a towel, toothbrush, or nailbrush with others.

When a handkerchief is soiled put it in water until it can be boiled (or, better still, use paper handkerchiefs and burn them when soiled).

Most important; wash the hands thoroughly before eating or handling food—and after using the lavatory. Keep finger-nails short and clean.

If in close contact with a new case of poliomyelitis, for three weeks afterwards keep at arm's length from other people; if possible sleep in a separate bed or, better still, in a separate room; avoid crowds and unnecessary travel; live in the fresh air as much as possible. See that children do not play with the children of other families. Avoid swimming baths, paddling pools, and crowds. If unwell rest and call the doctor.

In addition to carrying out these helpful injunctions issued by the council of the National Fund for Poliomyelitis Research it would be wise to give CAUSTICUM 30, three doses during a 24 hour period, to contacts as a preventive. This might well be followed three weeks later by three doses of LATHYRUS 30 given in the same way. This latter remedy has proved of value also in the treatment of this complaint.

Rheumatism

This somewhat vague term is employed as a convenient umbrella to cover a mort of mysteries. The term is met with in various forms such as muscular rheumatism (fibrositis), rheumatoid arthritis, monarticular rheumatism (osteoarthritis), rheumatic fever, even rheumatic gout. The cause, or causes, of rheumatism are elusive and the treatment often unsatisfactory. Some blame diet, others climate, or bacterial infection, or hypothetical toxins, or "acidity," or even failure of adaptation to stress.

From the practical point of view of treatment it must be realised that rheumatism is a highly individual matter. The homœopathic physician, with his individual approach to the patient as a whole, is, therefore, more likely to be able to help than the routinist.

The handling of a rheumatic condition in any form is a knotty medical problem, and from the homœopathic angle such remedies as those mentioned under the section on fibrositis will often prove of value if accurately prescribed. Various forms of physiotherapy intelligently employed under proper supervision have sometimes a part to play in alleviating pain and preventing stiffness, but internal homœopathic medication is the primary necessity.

Scarlet Fever—(see Sore Throat)

Septic Conditions

Prompt attention to cuts and abrasions as mentioned in the section on "Accidents" will often avoid septic inflammation. Where this is present from one cause or another the remedies referred to in the section on "Abscess" should be studied and the most "similar" given to speed the process of cure.

Skin Affections

It must be realised that the treatment of a so-called "skin disease" is in a great majority of cases a problem of internal medicine.

The skin is not only a protective covering well-equipped with sensory nerve endings as alarm signals, it is also a very important excretory organ and intimately associated with the well-being of the body as a whole. In many illnesses there is widespread disorder in the body and the skin shares in the disturbance. The skin eruption may be the most obvious symptom but the internal underlying disorder must be envisaged and dealt with if any cure is to be hoped for.

Consequently the cure of a skin trouble may be anything but straightforward, and the homœopathic physician with his approach to the patient as a whole and his method of individual investigation is well-equipped to deal with these complex problems.

A sensitive skin may, of course, be injured or irritated by direct contact with some chemical irritant, cosmetics, dyes, detergents, industrial chemicals, even medicaments applied with good intent or in response to fashion or popular acclaim. In this case the "fly in the ointment" must be sought out and avoided sedulously.

But more often the trouble is within and the skin disturbance is a response to internal irritants, food poisons, toxic drugs, autogenous toxins manufactured within the body, or to emotional stresses which upset the hormone balance and cause disorder in the circulation.

In general it is best to beware of ointments which often make matters worse by interfering with the excretory function of the skin. If the affected area is very dry and scaly pure olive oil may be applied. In the presence of a septic discharge a sterile dressing wrung out of HYPERICUM or CALENDULA lotion (ten drops of the mother tincture to the half pint of boiled water) may be used to cover the area. In intense irritation a similar lotion of HAMAMELIS (witch-hazel) may be applied for relief. But it is far better if possible to avoid all external applications, especially sulphur ointments or preparations of antibiotics, and attack the trouble from within.

As regards diet it will be necessary for the time-being to cut out sweets, especially chocolate, spicy foods, condiments, pastries, and indigestible things. It may be expedient to abstain from tea and coffee, also tobacco. Whole-meal bread and foods are to be preferred to bread and other eatables made with ordinary flour, which has been ruthlessly processed to the exclusion of essential ingredients and with the inclusion of substances of questionable value.

Each case must be studied individually and no hard and fast rules can be laid down as applicable to all alike. In some cases much patient perseverance is required for ultimate success.

Among the remedies of proven value in connection with skin affections may be mentioned the following (a few doses of 6 and the effect to be carefully watched):

ANTIMONIUM CRUDUM pustular eruptions (for instance, impetigo); corns, callosities, brittle nails, warts on hands (more prolonged treatment may be needed in these chronic conditions).

ARSENICUM ALBUM scaly eruptions which burn and itch.

GRAPHITES eruptions which exude a sticky fluid like honey; general dryness and roughness of the skin.

HEPAR SULPHURIS sores which fester easily and are excessively sensitive to least touch, even pressure of dressings, or to impact of cold air.

PETROLEUM eruptions which itch at night and ooze a thin watery discharge; tendency to cracks at finger tips and "chapped skin" in various sites.

RHUS TOXICODENDRON acute affections of skin which itch and burn and are associated with formation of blisters and local swelling.

SULPHUR much itching, worse from heat, and accompanied by irresistible desire to scratch.

Sore Throat

A sore throat must be treated with respect. It may be the herald or the concomitant of serious systemic disease, for instance diphtheria or scarlet fever, both of which carry additional risk of grave complications. Consequently the matter is one for expert medical investigation and care.

In case of contact with either of these infectious diseases it is wise to give the appropriate prophylactic remedy, DIPHTHERINUM or SCARLETINUM (three doses of 30 spread over the 24 hours) as both these infections has a short incubation period. Alternatively MERCURIUS CYANATUS 30, may be given to a diphtheria contact, or BELLADONNA 30 after the contact with scarlet fever (three doses as above).

There are a number of remedies intimately associated with various types of sore throat. The prompt administration of the most suitable remedy may avert serious illness, lessen the severity of an attack, and minimise the risk of complications.

The following are some of these (a dose of 30 every 4 to 6 hours for two or three days, if necessary, or 6 for a longer period two or three times daily):

ACONITUM burning, smarting, dryness, tingling in throat, which is very red; sudden onset after exposure to cold wind; fever and thirst for cold water; hurts to swallow.

APIS MELLIFICA burning, stinging pains in throat, which is swollen and soggy-looking; desire for coolth and **WORSE** heat; absence of thirst.

BARYTA CARBONICA sore throats developing slowly; recurrent tonsillitis; tendency to quinsy; tonsils and lymph nodes in neck enlarged.

BELLADONNA the typical scarlet fever throat—dry and burns like fire; fauces and tonsils inflamed and bright red; tongue bright red or "strawberry" appearance; spasm on trying to swallow so that food and fluids are ejected through mouth and nose; consequent aversion from taking fluids; red, hot face and skin, dilated pupils; tendency to violent delirium.

CAUSTICUM burning pain in throat, with soreness and rawness; throat feels constricted, must keep swallowing; hoarseness, relieved by coughing up mucus.

GELSEMIUM sore throat develops several days after exposure, in warm, moist, relaxing weather; difficulty in swallowing; cold shivers up and down back; lassitude, and heaviness all over; absence of thirst.

HEPAR SULPHURIS sore throat with well-established "cold"; sensation of fishbone or crumb stuck in throat; on swallowing pain shoots from throat into ears; throat extremely sensitive both within and without; pain in larynx on swallowing food; catarrhal swelling of pharynx with copious discharge; very irritable and sensitive to least cold draught.

LACHESIS soreness starts on left side, and later extends to right; throat looks bluish-red; feels as if closing up, or as if there was a lump causing a constant desire to swallow; much rawness and burning with a tendency to ulceration; can swallow solids better than fluids, in fact may get relief by taking solid food; cannot stand any pressure on throat, as from a tight collar.

MERCURIUS CYANATUS very severe type, with rapid onset, prostration, ulceration of fauces and membrane formation; thickly coated tongue; much salivation; putrid odour; hot sweats; tepid liquids swallowed better than either hot or cold. This remedy is of special avail in diphtheria.

MERCURIUS SOLUBILIS throat raw, sore, smarting; sore throat accompanies every "cold"; foul mouth; thirst despite moist mouth and much salivation; thick, yellow coating on tongue; throat feels dry and swallowing is painful, but must keep swallowing because of the free flow of saliva; is WORSE at night.

PHYTOLACCA throat sore, congested and dark red; throat feels full, as if would choke; every attempt to swallow sends pains shooting through ears; cannot swallow even water; sensation as if a ball of red-hot iron was stuck in throat; neck muscles feel stiff.

Toothache

There are a number of remedies which may give relief (a dose or two of 30 or 6 repeated at half-hourly intervals). If there is pain associated with a decayed hollow tooth a few drops of PLANTAGO mother tincture introduced into the cavity should relieve the pain.

ARNICA pain in tooth after "filling"; should be given also before and after tooth extraction.

BELLADONNA throbbing pain with dry mouth; gumboil.

CHAMOMILLA pain unbearable, aggravated by impact of cold air, also by taking anything warm into mouth and by drinking coffee.

COFFEA pain is aggravated by heat and hot fluids, and temporarily relieved by holding ice-cold water in mouth.

HEPAR SULPHURIS teeth very sensitive to touch; gums also sensitive and bleed easily.

MAGNESIA PHOSPHORICA neuralgic type of pain; somewhat relieved by heat and hot fluids; toothache during teething in children.

MERCURIUS teeth tender, loose, feel elongated; gums spongy, receding, bleed easily; alveolar abscess and pain WORSE at night; breath foul; thirsty despite excessive salivation.

PLANTAGO teeth ache and are sensitive to least touch; WORSE from contact with cold air; relief while eating; teeth feel too long; profuse flow of saliva.

PULSATILLA pain is unbearable; WORSE heat and hot fluids; BETTER by holding cold water in mouth; mouth dry, no thirst.

Travel Sickness

Many people get sick when travelling by car, boat or plane. There are probably two factors which may be responsible for this particularly disagreeable form of malaise. One is oxygen-lack resulting from lack of fresh air in a closed car, cabin, or railway compartment, possibly associated with pollution of the atmosphere by fumes. The other factor is the adverse effect on the organ of equilibrium in the ear of unusual motion. This tends to produce giddiness, headache, nausea and other symptoms.

Various patent medicines are advocated to "cure" this form of sickness and most of them depend on Hyoscine for their helpful effects. There are several remedies which, used homœopathically, have proved of value. The remedies (30 or 6) should be taken two or three times the day before starting and during the journey if required.

BORAX with its fear of downward motion, should be of value in air travel.

COCCULUS nausea associated with loathing, or even thought, of food, increased at sight or smell of food; inclination to vomit is accompanied by copious salivation; giddiness and unsteady gait; utter prostration and "all gone" hollow feeling; must lie down.

NUX VOMICA horrible queasy nausea, associated with splitting headache, often at back of head or over one eye, and loathing for food, tobacco, coffee; bloated feeling; much gagging, retching and rather ineffectual vomiting; wants warmth.

PETROLEUM persistent nausea with accumulation of water in mouth; pain in stomach with feeling of great emptiness and relief if something can be eaten; vomiting and giddiness which is WORSE from light or noise and on attempting to sit up; severe pain at back of head with stiffness of neck muscles; odd sensations in head.

RHUS TOXICODENDRON (especially of value in air sickness), nausea and vomiting accompanied by complete loss of appetite; extreme giddiness on attempting to rise; severe frontal headache; scalp sensitive to touch; mouth and throat dry, unquenchable thirst.

TABACUM nausea, giddiness, death-like pallor, vomiting, icy coldness, sweats, utter prostration; terrible faint sinking feeling; head feels gripped by a tight band; made WORSE by smell of tobacco smoke.

Warts

There are various kinds of wart or verruca, which is the Latin for wart. The remedy most often used, and frequently with success, is THUJA. The tincture should be painted on and the remedy given internally 6 twice a day, for a week or two at a time. ANTIMONIUM CRUDUM, CAUSTICUM or DULCAMARA may also be given internally in the same way.

Whooping-cough

This distressing malady is characterised by a peculiar kind of cough which comes on in relentless spasms. It is a machine-gun type of cough and at the end of the fit of coughing there may, or may not, be the well-known whoop. The latter is not necessarily present and it is important that the cough be recognised early and without waiting for the whoop to develop.

The remedy par excellence is DROSERA but on occasion others are indicated (a few doses of 30 for a day or two, or 6 for a longer period, three times a day):

BELLADONNA pain in stomach and tears precede the fit of coughing; throat gets drier and drier, then a violent tickle is followed by spasm of coughing, a whoop and gagging; a little mucus may be raised by great effort; cold aggravates.

BRYONIA starts a meal, takes a few mouthfuls, has a paroxysm of coughing, vomits, returns to finish the meal; springs up in bed with fit of coughing.

COCCUS CACTI is WORSE at night and from warmth of bed; is BETTER in a cool room and by taking cold drink; vomits tough ropy mucus.

DROSERA typical rapid-fire paroxysms; "crawling" sensation in throat; cough ends in vomiting; supports chest with hands.

This same remedy, DROSERA, may be used as a prophylactic for contacts, three doses of 30 being given during a 24 hour period.

INDEX

LIST OF REMEDIES MENTIONED IN TEXT

The 24 remedies in black type are of special value for emergency use.

The 30c potency is one of wide general use where only a few doses are called for.

A study of the text will show in what conditions a dose or two of a 200c may be of value; also when more prolonged treatment with 6c might be indicated.

Further information and literature, and names of chemists able to supply the medicines, can be obtained from the offices of the British Homœopathic Association.

ACONITUM NAPELLUS

AETHUSA CYNAPIUM

AGARICUS MUSCARIUS

ALLIUM CEPA

ALOE SOCOTRINA

ALUMINA

ANACARDIUM ORIENTALE

ANTHRACINUM

ANTIMONIUM CRUDUM

ANTIMONIUM TARTARICUM

APIS MELLIFICA

ARGENTUM NITRICUM

ARNICA MONTANA

ARSENICUM ALBUM

ARUM TRIPHYLLUM

BACILLINUM

BAPTISIA TINCTORIA

BARYTA CARBONICA

BELLADONNA

BERBERIS VULGARIS

BORAX

BRYONIA ALBA

CAJUPUTI

CALCAREA CARBONICA

CALENDULA OFFICINALIS

CAMPHORA

CANTHARIS VESICATORIA

CAPSICUM ANUUM

CARBO VEGETABILIS

CARBOLICUM ACIDUM

CAUSTICUM

CHAMOMILLA

CHINA OFFICINALIS

CICUTA VIROSA

CINA

COCCULUS INDICUS

COCCUS CACTI

COFFEA CRUDA

COLOCYNTHIS

CROTALUS HORRIDUS

CUPRUM ARSENICOSUM

CUPRUM METALLICUM

DIPHTHERINUM

DROSERA ROTUNDIFOLIA

DULCAMARA

ECHINACEA

EUPATORIUM PERFOLIATUM

EUPHRASIA OFFICINALIS

FERRUM PHOSPHORICUM

GELSEMIUM SEMPERVIRENS

GLONOINUM

GRAPHITES

HAMAMELIS VIRGINICA

HEPAR SULPHURIS CALCAREA

HYDRASTIS CANADENSIS
HYOSCYAMUS NIGER
HYPERICUM PERFOLIATUM

IGNATIA AMARA
INFLUENZINUM
IPECACUANHA

JABORANDI

KALI BICHROMICUM
KALI CARBONICUM
KALI IODATUM
KALI PHOSPHORICUM

LAC DEFLORATUM
LACHESIS MUTA
LATHYRUS SATIVA
LAUROCERASUS
LEDUM PALUSTRE
LYSSIN

MAGNESIA PHOSPHORICA
MEDUSA
MERCURIUS CORROSIVUS
MERCURIUS CYANATUS
MERCURIUS SOLUBILIS
MEZEREUM

NATRUM MURIATICUM
NATRUM SULPHURICUM
NICCOLUM METALLICUM
NUX VOMICA

OPIUM
OXALICUM ACIDUM

PAROTIDINUM
PETROLEUM
PHOSPHORUS

PHOSPHORICUM ACIDUM
PHYTOLACCA DECANDRA
PILOCARPINUM MURIATICUM
PLANTAGO MAJOR
PODOPHYLLUM PELTATUM
PULSATILLA NIGRICANS
PYROGENIUM

RANUNCULUS BULBOSUS
RHUS TOXICODENDRON
RUBELLA
RUMEX CRISPUS
RUTA GRAVEOLENS

SABADILLA
SCARLATININUM
SECALE CORNUTUM
SEPIA
SILICEA
SPIGELIA ANTHELMINTICA
SPONGIA TOSTA
STRAMONIUM
SULPHUR
SYMPHYTUM OFFICINALE

TABACUM
TAMUS COMMUNIS
TARANTULA CUBENSIS
THUJA OCCIDENTALIS

URTICA URENS

VERATRUM ALBUM
VERATRUM VIRIDE
VIBURNUM OPULUS
VIPERA TORVA

ZINCUM METALLICUM

The Association is a registered Charity supported entirely by men and women who, being convinced of the efficacy of the homoeopathic system of medicine, give regular subscriptions or donations for its maintenance. Applications for full details should be made to the Secretary, British Homoeopathic Association, 27a Devonshire Street, London W1N 1RJ.

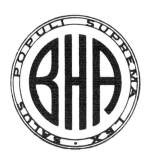

Homoeopathic Hospitals in the National Health Service

THE ROYAL LONDON HOMOEOPATHIC HOSPITAL,
Great Ormond Street, London, WC1N 3HR. Tel: 837 3091.

GLASGOW HOMOEOPATHIC HOSPITAL,
1000 Great Western Road, Glasgow, G12. Tel: 339 0382.

GLASGOW HOMOEOPATHIC OUT-PATIENT DEPARTMENT,
5 Lynedoch Crescent, Glasgow, G.3. Tel: 332 4490.

OUTPATIENT CLINIC FOR ADULTS & CHILDREN:
The Old Health Institute, Buchanan St, Baillieston, G69.
Tel. 041-771 7396

THE MOSSLEY HILL HOSPITAL — LIVERPOOL
(For Out and In Patients) Tel: 051-724-2335

BRISTOL HOMOEOPATHIC HOSPITAL,
Cotham, Bristol, 6. Tel: Bristol 731231

TUNBRIDGE WELLS HOMOEOPATHIC HOSPITAL,
Church Road, Tunbridge Wells. Tel: Tunbridge Wells 0892 42977

THE MANCHESTER CLINIC,
Brunswick Street, Ardwick, Manchester. Tel: 061-273-2446
(This Clinic is NOT N.H.S.)

© British Homoeopathic Association